The Essential Oils Menopause Solution

Also by Dr. Mariza Snyder

The Essential Oils Hormone Solution

Smart Mom's Guide to Essential Oils

The DASH Diet Cookbook (with Lauren Clum and Anna V. Zulaica)

The Matcha Miracle (with Lauren Clum and Anna V. Zulaica)

Water Infusions (with Lauren Clum)

The Lo-GI Slow Cooker (with Lauren Clum and Anna V. Zulaica)

The Antioxidant Counter (with Lauren Clum)

The Essential Oils Menopause Solution

Alleviate Your Symptoms and Reclaim Your Energy, Sleep, Sex Drive, and Metabolism

Dr. Mariza Snyder

RODALE BOOKS

NEW YORK

No book can replace the diagnostic expertise and medical advice of a trusted physician. Please be certain to consult with your doctor before making any decisions that affect your health, particularly if you suffer from any medical conditions or have any symptoms that may require treatment.

Library of Congress Cataloging-in-Publication Data
Names: Snyder, Mariza, author.
Title: The essential oils menopause solution : alleviate your symptoms and reclaim your energy, sleep, sex drive, and metabolism / Dr. Mariza Snyder.
Description: New York : Rodale Books [2021] | Includes bibliographical references and index.
Identifiers: LCCN 2020033914 (print) | LCCN 2020033915 (ebook) | ISBN 9780593137093 (hardcover) | ISBN 9780593137109 (epub)
Subjects: LCSH: Menopause—Alternative treatment. | Essences and essential oils. | Self-care, Health.
Classification: LCC RG186 .S697 2021 (print) | LCC RG186 (ebook) | DDC 618.1/75--dc23
LC record available at https://lccn.loc.gov/2020033914
LC ebook record available at https://lccn.loc.gov/2020033915

ISBN 978-0-593-13709-3
Ebook ISBN 978-0-593-13710-9

Printed in the United States of America

Jacket design by Anna Bauer
Jacket photograph by Hitdelight/Shutterstock

10 9 8 7 6 5 4 3 2 1

First Edition

FOR MY HUSBAND, ALEX,
who brings joy to my life each day and who
knows almost as much as I do about women's
hormone health. Thank you for your endless
support, delicious taco dinners, and keeping
life sweet and full of laughter.

Contents

PART III

The 21-Day Hormone Makeover Program

Introduction

More than once, you've likely heard doctors, family members, and friends say that it's completely normal to feel a little tired, stressed, and moody, especially near your period or as you approach menopause. Feeling this way is so normal, in fact, there is nothing you can do to make yourself feel better—except pop a pill to manage the symptoms. As an adult woman in today's modern world, you just have to grit your teeth and wait it out, hoping somehow your symptoms go away.

That is a big fat lie. What you are experiencing *isn't normal.*

There is no objective reason why you should feel terrible during perimenopause and menopause. Yes, as your ovarian function declines and your hormone levels shift, your body will change—there's no getting around that. But it is a natural, normal process your body was designed to navigate. You can and should experience optimal health during this time, including a good night's sleep, clear thinking, stable moods, and pain-free sex. No matter what your age, you always deserve a body that works for you, and if you are feeling less than your best, you deserve solutions that promote actual healing.

Unfortunately, many doctors, even gynecologists, cannot tell you the difference between perimenopause and menopause or how to treat the myriad of symptoms most women experience during this time of change. And too often they default to treating symptoms with a prescription pad or dismissing them as natural signs of growing older. Women are still regularly told that exhaustion, sleeplessness, brain fog, low libido, hot flashes, weight gain, and headaches are inevitable with age.

I know you've noticed troubling changes to your mood, sleep, digestion, weight, and, if you are still menstruating, your cycle. You're probably cursing your hormones, namely that darn estrogen, and struggling to get through each day. You may have even been to a doctor who waved off your symptoms, telling you everything is normal and you are just experiencing natural signs of aging.

Or, maybe a doctor told you the only way to feel better is to pop a pill to manage the symptoms: take the birth control pill, bioidentical hormones, or an antidepressant to ease your discomfort.

But there is more you can do. There are lifestyle changes, supplementation protocols, and self-care rituals—including many that incorporate essential oils—that will help you get at the root cause and find balance for all of the hormones playing a role in your symptoms. I am not just talking about your reproductive hormones. I am also referring to your hormones that control your metabolism, stress response, cognitive function, mood, sleep, digestion, hunger, hair growth, and much more.

You are a superwoman. But if you've picked up this book, I know you are feeling less-than, defeated, and worried. You probably have several of the symptoms I've mentioned earlier. I want you to know: You are not alone! We are in this together. You are the CEO of your own healthcare, and *you* can naturally restore balance to your hormones and your life. With foundational lifestyle habits including proper nutrition, supplementation, movement, and self-care incorporating the regular use of essential oils, we can reset our hormones, restore health, and transition into perimenopause and beyond with ease and grace—and without debilitating symptoms or medication.

The "Why" Behind This Book: Mom's Story

I remember the night my mom finally reached out for help, just like you are doing now. The phone rang late at night, waking me up and startling me. I could hear the fear and defeat in her voice, a tone I have rarely ever heard from her my entire life.

As a single mother, my mom, Jody, battled in the trenches to raise my sister Cynthia and me. We struggled for years to get by in a small two-bedroom apartment, though we didn't realize how much our mom endured until years later. The stress and exhaustion of single motherhood took its toll, but she always persevered. She made such an impression on me that I always wanted to be just like her when I grew up. Graduating from college at age twenty-seven, she built an incredible career to show her girls how to succeed. She fought for us constantly, and I always admired her: her polished look, her determined demeanor, the intentional way she approached life. She made the impossible possible.

But, as things tend to do when we neglect ourselves, my mom began to show signs of falling apart. She continually drove herself into the ground, the chronic rush wearing her down day by day until someone we didn't recognize began to show up at home. In a Jekyll-and-Hyde-type switch, she would turn into a woman who flew off the handle, causing us to hide in another room until the bubbly, giggling, empowered mama that we loved surfaced from the darkness again. With the benefit of my medical training, I now know that she was struggling with intense hormonal imbalances. But there was one thing I always knew to be true. My mom always loved us, even when she struggled, even when severe PMS derailed her emotionally and physically. We may not have understood what was going on inside her body and could only react to the outward manifestations of these intense hormonal issues, but we knew she loved us.

Her hormonal fluxes only worsened with age. Shocked and overwhelmed by the intensity of her anger, she still went nuclear over minor inconveniences until one day at age thirty-nine she let loose on a stranger who had blocked her driveway. She could feel that stress, irritability, and the I'm-gonna-snap-if-one-more-thing-happens feeling building up inside, but she charged on thinking if she could just get home and relax it would all go away for a moment. She shocked herself that day, and that was the turning point. She knew something wasn't right inside of her and she needed help.

But guess what? Even after mustering up the courage to make a doctor's appointment, to go in and confess all the embarrassing symptoms, and to be so openly vulnerable as to ask, "Is it normal to want to kill someone during your period?," she got the usual response. The doctor responded, "Yes, it can be." Which is an utter lie. Nothing about what my mom was experiencing was normal.

The doctor did one good thing for my mom; she validated her symptoms. But in letting her know she wasn't alone, she also committed the giant mistake of normalizing her symptoms. There is *nothing* normal about them. And she didn't understand that there were root causes driving all of her intense symptoms. Normalizing our symptoms doesn't create hormone balance. It might make us feel a little less alone, but who wants to suffer silently together?

But it gave my mama the bump she needed to soldier on until her late forties, when her hormones took a severe nose dive. Erratic sleep, inexplicable weight gain, severe fatigue, and exhaustion by 4 p.m. consumed her every single day. She pushed through, accepting this as her new normal based on the confidence the doctor had given her. Then the irregular periods began, followed by severe heavy bleeding and hot flashes leaving her drenched in sweat at work in the operating room.

"It must be menopause," she reasoned. And she charged on until hot flashes lit her up multiple times a week and her thin frame carried twenty-five extra pounds. Until insomnia and fatigue pulled her into a tired-and-wired cycle, and the worry crept back in again.

What's a woman in perimenopause to do? My mom reached out to a women's hormone practice in search for solutions—without my knowledge. She knew enough to request blood work on her reproductive, stress, and thyroid hormones, but this doctor told her those tests weren't reliable and so didn't use them. Instead of digging deeper into root causes, the doctor pulled out a prescription pad and offered her an "easy fix": an estrogen patch. Mom was so desperate for relief that she was willing to try anything.

The hormone therapy worked for a couple of weeks, relieving her of hot flashes during her workday, but the rest of her symptoms persisted and new ones began to appear that she had never, *ever* experienced before. In two months' time, she suffered from more weight gain, chronic headaches, and intense insomnia coupled with bone-crushing fatigue. This "easy fix" dropped her into a circle of hell and kept pushing her in deeper and deeper.

It got worse. Depression began to impact her motivation and drive. She withdrew from life, with zero motivation to work out or to hang out with friends—and eventually even to function.

My mom was scared of these new symptoms and didn't know where to turn.

And that is when she called me, embarrassed, desperate, and incredibly freaked out. The fear in her voice pulsed as she told me the details. The last thing she said was in a whisper: "I'm starting to have scary thoughts . . ."

Despite my immediate fear and concern for my mom, I got her to a safe place and, after a long conversation, assured her that she would be okay. That I would not rest until we figured this out. Over the next weeks, I worked with her to slowly wean her off the estrogen patch and then ran a full panel of hormone tests to check thyroid hormones, stress hormones, all reproductive hormones, plus DHEA, insulin, and other important markers (see The Importance of Testing on page 284 for my testing recommendations). She also immediately started my Hormone Makeover Protocol, the basis of the 21-Day Hormone Makeover Program that you will find in part III of this book. I also recommended key essential oils to help support her hot flashes, insomnia, fatigue, and depressed feelings. She carried these powerful, simple solutions on her at all times, especially when she needed an instant pick-me-up.

Within thirty days, my mom's depression lifted, she lost eighteen pounds, and she was waking up early with energy to work and play tennis. Emotionally, she began to feel like herself again. By day 60, she called to tell me that she felt like a younger version of herself. "I honestly didn't think I could feel this way again! It's like I was given my body back and I feel on top of the world. If this is what midlife actually feels like, sign me up!" she gushed. "I've lost twenty-five pounds. I am not tired in the afternoon anymore. I don't have crazy soda cravings anymore, and I feel so much happier. My motivation is in full swing and my hair and skin feel and look healthier. I honestly feel like myself at thirty-seven years old, especially without the hot flashes. I am ready for life to bring it on."

And there she was again, my Warrior Mama.

I allowed myself to exhale for a minute before the warrior woman inside of me became supercharged with determination. It was time to empower other women and get them all back on track. To get *you* back on track. If my mom could turn back time on her health, I knew every woman could too by tapping into the healing potential inside her. We just need to figure out the right way to do it for each individual.

This is *exactly* why I began writing this book.

Reclaim Your Energy, Radiance, and Healthcare—How to Use This Book

Ideally, perimenopause and menopause should be a natural transition that sets you up for a brand-new phase in your life. The best way to naturally support your body through midlife and menopause is by getting your body functioning effectively on a cellular level through your daily habits, aided every step of the way by:

- **Essential oils:** Able to quickly and effectively calm, uplift, ground, and/or energize, essential oils support the body's healing potential at the cellular level.
- **Plant-focused nutrition:** Eating food that works for you, nourishing your body with all of the nutrients it needs to thrive, will ensure that your body gets back into balance and stays there.

- **Movement:** By incorporating regular movement that makes your body and soul happy, you'll strengthen and support your muscles, improve mental focus, and reduce stress while supporting hormone balance.
- **Self-care rituals:** Finding ways to care for yourself, from the inside out, will not only help put your body back in balance but allow you to support everyone and everything else in your life better.
- **Supplementation:** If you are struggling with hormone imbalances, it can be really difficult to get the key nutrients you need from food alone. That's where supplements come in.

Though prescribing medications and hormones may seem like an easy solution, oftentimes they can obstruct your ability to truly heal and create longevity. Getting to the root cause of perimenopause and menopause symptoms takes some time, but this book will give you a step-by-step system to support your hormones and leave you feeling energized, joyful, and revitalized.

Spotlight: Supplements

Pure, well-crafted supplements can step in and bridge the nutritional gaps to jump-start your journey to healing and balance. The problem is that many supplements are of low quality and not effective, or bioavailable, meaning they simply don't work. Over the last decade I have extensively researched the quality, bioavailability, and efficacy of many supplements for hormone pathways and cellular support. As a biochemist and functional practitioner, I took extra steps to understand how specific supplements are created and tested for purity. Nothing I found on the market met my quality standards, so I created my own line: Essentially Whole®.

Each Essentially Whole® supplement has been carefully chosen or formulated by me and includes highly absorbable, bioavailable ingredients painstakingly researched and carefully selected. Tested for purity and efficacy, they are all gluten free, dairy free, GMO free, soy free, corn free, and free of any harmful fillers and flavors. I scrutinize how my supplements are formulated and tested, even going to the facility where they are created to observe each and every step in the quality control and testing process.

I also take them each and every day myself, and have been astounded by the results physiologically and in my lab results. I encourage you to try them out and share your amazing results with me.

In Part I, What's Going On with My Hormones in Menopause, you will learn what hormones are, what their roles are in your body, how they become unbalanced, and the key root causes driving hormone imbalance. Then we'll start talking solutions, covering the scientific basis of how essential oils work from a physiological aspect to reset and improve hormonal levels, the specific therapeutic properties of the oils most commonly used to address hormonal symptoms, which essential oils are best to support perimenopause and menopause, and everything you need to know to start using essential oils right away. Knowing the science and understanding how your body works will give you the power to move forward into this next phase of life.

Part II, Using Nutrition, Supplementation, Essential Oils, and Natural Remedies to Address Your Perimenopausal and Menopausal Symptoms, is organized by topic, so you can quickly turn to the chapter or chapters addressing an issue you're dealing with. The solutions you'll find in these chapters are designed to work with your unique biochemistry, and will help you anticipate potential issues and symptoms. We will work to banish the worst symptoms of perimenopause and menopause, including minimizing hot flashes and boosting your libido. Easing these symptoms will in turn improve your energy and mood and strengthen your focus and concentration. Anticipating what your body needs will help you gain the confidence to move into your future on your terms.

With more than seventy-five recipes for essential oil blends created specifically for this book, you will be able to easily locate and implement specific solutions for your individualized needs. Plus, they are so incredibly easy to make and use, your friends may start begging you for your Hot Flash Extinguisher Spritz and I've Got This Rollerball Blend.

Part III, The 21-Day Hormone Makeover Program, is the ultimate solution to resetting your hormones and drastically improving your health and longevity. Adapting your lifestyle to balance your hormones can be easy with the plan I have carefully created for you. I'll get you ready with daily solutions and amazing self-care rituals before you start, so you'll be ready and fully supported during the step-by-step program with meal plans, exercise recommendations, recipes, supplement protocols, and effective essential oils for the following three weeks. You will be astonished by how much better you will feel, and how easy it is to incorporate healthy choices into your life for a powerful transformation with lasting results.

More than 130 years ago, a woman's life expectancy was forty years. Now, in the United States, our average life expectancy is eighty-three years. No longer is midlife an end or a time of sickness, inactivity, and invisibility. It's the beginning of an opportunity to soar into the second half of our lives with grace, vitality, confidence, and the personal and professional wisdom gained from our earlier life experiences. Balanced hormones are the foundation of an extraordinary, vibrant life and this book is designed to show you step by step how to make it happen.

And how do I know this is possible? My mom did it. And she didn't just reclaim her life; she reinvented it based on what she loved. She decided to take on marathon running shortly after her hormone makeover, and since then she has run more than seventy marathon and half-marathon races. And you know she has the medals to prove it! Today, my mom is rocking her life with confidence, grace, and high energy.

If You Are on the Birth Control Pill or Hormone Therapy

If you have picked up this book and you are currently on birth control pills or hormone therapy, I want you to know that you are in the right place. Whether you are taking hormones to manage your symptoms or not, this book will provide safe, effective natural solutions and lifestyle changes that you can implement while taking hormone therapy. They will also support you if you are transitioning off hormones or are interested in doing so in the future.

The Time Is Now

My mother's story inspired me to write this book, but every day I field questions from other women who are in similar situations—women who suspect that there is more to their hormonal story than "just normal aging" and who are desperate for solutions that their own doctors are not providing. I want you to know that I hear you. I hear that you feel invisible, dismissed, neglected, and unsupported. I hear that you are confused and overwhelmed with misinformation. I hear that you are struggling without clear solutions. With this book, I hope to validate you and answer you with straightforward, science-backed replies to your most frequent questions and concerns and provide you with solutions that work. I also want to flip the script on fear.

My mom, Jody, allowed me to be her advocate. And that's what we all need. An advocate. A healthcare team. The confidence to be our own kind of superwoman.

Let me be your advocate and support you every step of the way. My hope is that the information, encouragement, practical advice, and step-by-step protocol in this book empower you with the confidence to take charge of your healthcare and transform your life.

You can turn back time on your health and redefine midlife on your terms.

You can reclaim your sleep and wake up feeling rested and ready to charge.

You can rebalance your hormones to rid your life of monthly-cycle hell.

You can cultivate longevity and vitality.

You can saunter gracefully into menopause, embracing life without horrible symptoms.

The next chapters of your life can be the best yet. Join me by turning the page and we will revolutionize your body together.

PART I

What's Going On with My Hormones in Menopause

Chapter 1

Understanding Your Reproductive Hormones

"Why am I exhausted all the time?"

"Why am I always so stressed out?"

"Why can't I sleep through the night anymore?"

"Why can't I lose this weight around my middle? I'm exercising and eating like I always have!"

"Why can't I remember anything? Why is my mind so cloudy?"

"What the heck is going on?!"

Hormones!

Hormones are chemical messengers that regulate most everything that happens in your body: appetite, metabolism, hair growth, sleep, body temperature, mood, sex drive, and menstruation. The female hormones of estrogen and progesterone play starring roles in our reproductive cycles, so it's no surprise they get top billing during puberty, when we transition into our fertile years, and perimenopause and menopause, as we stop getting our periods. But they aren't onstage alone. There is a whole cast of hormones that play a critical part in your health and well-being during both these transitional times as well as every single day in between.

Because our body's systems are so interconnected, hormones work together in a sort of grand symphony to maintain a harmonious balance and keep everything running optimally. If one hormone goes off-script, other hormones are thrown off balance—throwing you off balance. But it is precisely this complexity that makes it nearly impossible to isolate one hormone as responsible for all of our problems. Instead, we must look at the interplay of a variety of them.

That's why it's so important for you to understand some hormone basics. With a clear grasp of what your hormones do and how they fluctuate, especially before, during, and after menopause, you'll see that none of the symptoms you are experiencing are random or coming out of nowhere. There are reasons why you're feeling like you do based on your own specific chemistry, your past and present experiences, your lifestyle choices, and your environment. The good news is that we can anticipate these changes and symptoms, and adapt your lifestyle to find solutions that work specifically for your needs.

Let's start connecting the dots with a closer look at the nonadolescent hormonal changes: perimenopause, menopause, and the dubious new term, "postmenopause."

What's Perimenopause?

The quick answer: an unpredictable time of transition. The truth is that most people mistake perimenopause for menopause, not realizing the distinction between the two. "Peri" means "around" or "about," so any time before your period has been gone for one solid year falls within the perimenopause spectrum. It can start as early as your mid to late thirties and last anywhere from four to twelve years.

During perimenopause, you still have periods even if they become irregular. This means you can still get pregnant. But know that estrogen levels fluctuate rapidly, spiking up and down as the ovaries begin to slack off in production. Some women breeze through perimenopause, while others experience a spectrum of hormone fluctuations so wild and erratic that they cause a wide range of undesirable changes: hot flashes, night sweats, sleep problems, severe PMS, heavy bleeding, memory issues, vaginal dryness, fatigue, and brain fog, among others. Perimenopause can be enormously disruptive physically and emotionally, but it doesn't have to be. The goal is for you to prepare for the worst, but adapt for the best!

Perimenopause is a natural phase of life. Your body is beautifully designed to wind down at a certain point, giving you a release from reproduction. Your body is also unique to you and there is no way to predict exactly how it will respond to these hormone changes. But I see perimenopause coming on earlier and more intensely for many women because so many of us are completely stressed and burned out. In putting others before ourselves, we delay self-care, contributing to widespread hormone imbalance and inflammation—and a rocky perimenopause.

The most important thing to remember is that your body is supposed to go through this natural, biological change, and you can control how you prepare and respond. Supporting and nurturing your body during this time by prioritizing self-care and a lifestyle that supports hormone balance offers you the best chance for an easy, graceful transition. Just ask my mom!

The Truth About the Options for Easing Your Way Through Perimenopause

The Pill for Perimenopause Symptoms

You can fix hormone imbalance without adding hormones. You do *not* need the pill or any form of hormonal contraceptive to ease your symptoms. The pill and other forms of hormonal birth control (the patch, vaginal ring, shot, injection, implant, or hormonal IUD) are *contraceptives,* intended to be used to prevent pregnancy. Yet, a lot of doctors would have you think they do even more, such as "fix" painful or heavy periods, PMS or PMDD (premenstrual dysphoric disorder), and irregular or missing periods. In fact, the majority of American women on the birth control pill, a whopping 58 percent, take it for reasons other than preventing pregnancy. Here's the truth. They don't solve these issues; they mask them by adding synthetic estrogen and progesterone to your body, preventing it from functioning the way it was designed. While these synthetic hormones may temporarily hide symptoms, your body has to work harder to overcome their effect. And that is why new symptoms begin to appear: migraines, decreased libido, vaginal dryness, abnormal uterine bleeding and spotting, thyroid dysfunction, blood clots and deep vein thrombosis, anxiety and depression, and the list continues. So, you may find symptom relief by staying on the pill or starting to take it during perimenopause, but you have to be aware of the side effects and the fact that you are not addressing the real causes for your symptoms. This is why I want you to know: Natural solutions like the ones covered in this book will relieve symptoms by addressing the root cause of the problem without scary, unnecessary side effects.

In some cases, if natural solutions are not working as well as hoped, the pill may be considered to provide a short-term solution to severe symptoms, helping you regain your equilibrium. But as a functional practitioner, I always encourage trying natural options first.

Endometrial Ablation for Heavy Bleeding During Perimenopause

Endometrial ablation is an outpatient procedure that cauterizes (ablates) the lining of the uterus (endometrium) in order to prevent growth and future bleeding. Doctors can use a variety of techniques to achieve this end; I prefer the NovaSure procedure, which uses radiofrequency. In certain situations, I do agree that endometrial ablation can be a viable option. For example, when a woman has developed anemia that can't be successfully reversed due to extreme bleeding, all other options such as supplementation and/or lifestyle changes have been exhausted, and she has decided that she is done reproducing.

What worries me is that endometrial ablation seems to be the new "facelift for your uterus" procedure that middle-aged women are electing to have simply because they are tired of their periods. It's even touted by some doctors as "one of the great gynecological success stories" for reducing menstrual flow. You need to understand that heavy bleeding during perimenopause is *not* abnormal, due to sporadic ovulation and increased estrogen levels. When your body doesn't release an egg, the endometrium continues to grow, causing the next period to be heavier than previous ones. This is *normal*.

I understand the allure of not having to slink off to the bathroom to recover from leaking pads or tampons, and that ditching the crampy, achy menstrual mess each month would be a relief. But please be sure that you have tried everything else to firm up your foundation—diet, exercise, supplements, stress management, self-care—to address estrogen dominance and hormonal imbalance before jumping off the deep end into a procedure that cannot be reversed. (For more on heavy bleeding, see Chapter 14.)

What's Menopause?

Menopause is the complete absence of any menstrual bleeding for at least one year.

It's as simple as that. Once you've gone twelve consecutive months without a period, you are in menopause. The hormonal roller-coaster ride of perimenopause ends. Your ovaries stop producing estrogen and progesterone and cease to release an egg each month (ovulation). And now it's official: Your body is done making babies. It won't continue to prime you each month to do so. You remain in menopause for the rest of your life; it's a permanent state of being. Menopause presents our bodies with an opportunity to rest from reproduction and use that energy elsewhere! Menopause is the start of a new beginning.

So, how will you know you're in menopause? The onset doesn't happen like it does on television. You don't just wake up one day covered with sweat, sobbing into your floral comforter. Menopause is a journey along the road of life.

The only for-sure factor is that you haven't menstruated for a full year's time. There isn't a hormone test to determine when that will happen, though some healthcare providers will measure your FSH, or follicle-stimulating hormone, levels through either blood or saliva to try to do so. Your FSH levels will reach their peak in menopause, but they can also become elevated in perimenopause, so this one test alone isn't reliable. It's a waiting game, and that is hard, especially when erratic periods can get your hopes up.

The average age of natural menopause is fifty-one, but there are no hard and fast rules here. Some women naturally enter menopause in their early forties, while others don't until their late fifties. Many women bank on the age of their mother's onset as their telltale marker, but many, many factors contribute to this change.

There are other forms of menopause that you could experience, but most have outside factors that force their hand. Premature menopause can happen before the age of forty, and is usually linked to an illness or a preexisting condition, though chronic stress can be a cause, too. Artificial menopause (also called surgical or chemical menopause) is brought on by the removal of both ovaries; for example, in a hysterectomy, or disruption of the blood supply to the ovaries because of radiation, chemotherapy, or drugs. Artificial menopause comes on immediately and usually much stronger than natural menopause. But, for most women, we just wait and trust our body to find its natural rhythm.

The good news about menopause is that the wild hormonal ride of perimenopause is over. The bad news is that you may still be experiencing the same perimenopause symptoms you had been dealing with or noticing new ones. The reason: You're still burned out! Your symptoms are *not* always tied to your ovaries and an estrogen deficiency, but rather widespread hormonal havoc rooted in stress and less-than-stellar lifestyle habits. In fact, too much estrogen—including estrogen stored in your fatty tissues—could still be causing some of your symptoms. *Those hormonal imbalances* are driving the mood swings, migraines, disrupted sleep, fatigue, and other symptoms hastily misunderstood and tagged as "menopause." But guess what? If you get a handle on a healthy foundational lifestyle and understand what's happening, you get a handle on those symptoms. In fact, you can even anticipate their arrival and adapt right now to ease your body into these natural changes.

Menopause is usually considered a dirty word or a condition that needs to be treated. Listen to me when I tell you this: It's neither. Our amazing bodies are designed for menopause to happen when our reproductive years are over, and if we support them with a good foundation, we should be able to gracefully saunter into our next phase of life with confidence, knowing that we have done everything in our power to adapt and support our bodies.

Redefining Menopause

It's a common misnomer that menopause means you are officially old. That it is the end of your vitality, beauty, femininity, sexuality, and passion. Please. The only thing menopause ends is your ability to make a baby. Period.

Let me be realer than real: The feminine body is a miracle. The ability to conceive, nurture, and nourish a child is just one of the many miracles we were designed to do. Think about all of the other complex biological functions it executes every single day, and you can rest assured that your estrogen level doesn't dictate your vitality. Here are just a few examples of what menopause really means.

Freedom from periods. No more anxiety over planning around your cycle. No more missed life experiences because of cramps or heavy flow. No more pants ruined because of leaks.

Postmenopausal zest. Renowned anthropologist Margaret Mead coined this term in response to an ageist/sexist comment by a talk-show host who had questioned her ability to achieve a breadth of work that would have exhausted someone half her age, to which she retorted, "It might have killed me too at that age. I attribute my energy to postmenopausal zest." Yes! Now that your body isn't spending its energy focusing on reproduction each month, it has energy to spare.

Hormonal rebalance. During perimenopause, your reproductive hormones are on a roller-coaster ride. Once you reach menopause, your reproductive hormones will stabilize, easing some of the symptoms you may have been experiencing during perimenopause.

Reinventing yourself. With reproduction off your plate and symptoms easing, menopause offers the opportunity to focus on you. It is time to inventory your needs and identify what brings you joy. Once upon a time, when women's life expectancy was significantly shorter, menopause may have occurred at the "end" of life. But now, as we're living longer and well into our eighties and beyond, menopause truly is midlife. Spend the next few decades happy, empowered, and thriving.

What's Postmenopause?

"Postmenopause" is the new trendy term used to refer to the period of time after twelve months have passed since your last period. ("Post" means "after.") Those who use this term think of it like this:

Perimenopause (*before menopause*)

↓

Menopause (*the moment you've gone twelve months without a period*)

↓

Postmenopause (*after menopause*)

The trouble is, "postmenopause" is a redundant term. By its very definition, "menopause" is a permanent state of being that covers this time of life. We don't need another word to describe these years. I prefer to be straightforward with my science. If your reproductive years are over, everything in this book for women in menopause applies to you.

The Role of Reproductive Hormones

Whether or not you are still capable of reproducing, your reproductive hormones always matter. They support your total physical and emotional health, not just your sexual development and reproduction. Below is a rundown of the star players, the ones that change over time and more significantly (and naturally) during perimenopause and menopause. I've broken it down into basics for you, also giving you signs that you might have too much or too little, and what to expect during menopause. If you suspect imbalances of any of these, take note now, as you will definitely learn how to support them as we progress in this book.

DHEA, or dehydroepiandrosterone, is a hormone produced primarily by your adrenal glands that converts into the reproductive hormones estrogen and testosterone. DHEA production peaks in your midtwenties and slows with age. Too much DHEA can result in polycystic ovarian syndrome (PCOS), excess hair growth on the face and body (hirsutism), hair loss, irregular menstruation, infertility, acne, Cushing's disease, congenital adrenal hyperplasia, adrenal cancer, or tumors. Having too little DHEA is also problematic. It can result in Addison's disease, dementia, diabetes, low libido, osteoporosis, chronic fatigue syndrome, autoimmune diseases such as lupus and Hashimoto's disease, and vaginal atrophy or dryness.

Estrogen is a catchall word for any compound that produces estrus. We typically focus on the three most important ones when referring to "estrogen" as a whole: estrone, estradiol, and estriol. These three hormones drive the growth and development of a woman's body, including breasts and other secondary sex characteristics, as well as bone density. They also regulate the menstrual cycle, and assist in practically every physiological function. That's right. Your heart, brain, bones, bladder, colon, and practically every other organ in your body relies on estrogen to work properly. During our fertile years, estrogens are produced primarily in the ovaries. In menopause, the ovaries no longer produce estrogen and instead they come mainly from adipose (fat) tissue. Let's take a closer look at the three main estrogens:

Estrone (E1), also known as oestrone, is produced by the ovaries and adrenal glands, as well as our fat tissue (the more fat, the more estrone), and it is responsible for our sexual development and functioning. Because it is less active than estradiol, estrone can be converted into estradiol when necessary. Too much estrone is linked to breast cancer and endometrial cancer growth. Too little is linked to osteoporosis and menopause symptoms, such as hot flashes, decreased libido, fatigue, and depression.

Estrone is the most dominant estrogen during menopause.

Estradiol (E2), also known as oestradiol, is the everyday powerhouse player of the three types of estrogen. Produced directly in the ovaries, estradiol rules in our reproductive system, maturing and maintaining the entire operation. During the menstrual cycle, rising levels cause an egg to mature and release (ovulation) and stimulate the thickening of the uterine lining for successful implantation. Estradiol levels decrease during pregnancy, but increase postgestation. Levels do lower with age, with the most significant decline at menopause when the ovaries stop producing it and we will get it solely from adipose (fat) tissue.

Having too much estradiol can lead to acne, constipation, decreased libido, depression, and weight gain. In extremely high levels, it is implicated in uterine and breast cancer and cardiovascular disease. Having too little estradiol can hinder bone growth and development and delay puberty, as well as accelerate osteoporosis, insulin resistance, and increase mood swings.

Estriol (E3), also known as oestriol, is the pregnancy estrogen, released in mass quantities by the placenta. It's almost undetectable in women who are not pregnant.

External Estrogens: The Good, the Bad, and the Ugly

In addition to the estrogens created by your body, you should be aware of the "foreign" estrogens present in our environment. These are so close in molecular structure to natural estrogen that they can compete with our hormones for estrogen receptors. (A hormone receptor is like a lock guarding entry to the cell, and its matching hormone is the key to opening it.) Simply put, some external estrogens are good and some are not.

The Good: Phytoestrogens

Phytoestrogens are estrogenic compounds naturally found in fruits and veggies, legumes, and some grains. In our bodies, they function like estrogen, binding with estrogen receptors, but are estimated to be 500 to 1,000 times weaker than what our bodies produce naturally. They are also adaptogenic and can help to support our bodies when natural levels run too low or too high. For this reason, phytoestrogens are often used to lessen the symptoms brought on by perimenopause and menopause.

The Bad and the Ugly: Xenoestrogens and Synthetics

These two are known as endocrine disruptors, and they wreak havoc on your hormones and your body. They are both man-made. **Xenoestrogens** such as BPA, parabens, and phthalates are found in everything from your personal and beauty care products to shopping receipts. **Synthetic estrogens** are those produced by the pharmaceutical industry and are found in the birth control pill and hormone therapy.

Progesterone is the "see" to estrogen's "saw," balancing out estrogen's type-A personality. Produced in the ovaries during menstruation, the placenta during pregnancy, and the adrenal glands during menopause, progesterone is best known for maintaining the safe, cushy lining of the uterus to help a fertilized egg grow. But it does so much more! Progesterone helps us use fat for energy, maintain normal thyroid function and blood sugar levels, restore libido, and lower our risk for certain types of cancer. In addition, it's a natural antidepressant, anxiety reliever, and diuretic, preventing water retention and swelling. In menopause, your progesterone levels are naturally very low, since you are no longer menstruating. During menopause, if you have too much progesterone, you may experience weight gain, fatigue, breast tenderness, bloating, mood swings, depression, and digestive issues. If you have too little, you may have irregular menstrual cycles, infertility, a high risk of miscarriage or preterm delivery, spotting, vaginal dryness, PMS, low libido, anxiety, and headaches or migraines.

Testosterone isn't just for men. We women rely on this hormone, which is produced in the ovaries and adrenal glands, for bone health, muscle development, and to keep our sex drive humming. Testosterone levels peak in your twenties and decline slowly with age. In menopause, the ovaries continue to make testosterone, as do the adrenal glands, but its level is half of what it was at its peak. Too much testosterone leads to irregular menstrual cycles, excessive or thinning hair, changes in mood, acne, low libido, and excess hair growth on the face, back, and chest (hirsutism). Too little also leads to irregular menstrual cycles and low libido but also muscle weakness, fatigue, loss of bone density, and vaginal dryness.

FSH (follicle-stimulating hormone) is true to its name, stimulating the ovarian follicles, fluid-filled sacs that contain immature eggs, to mature and produce estrogen. Made in the pituitary gland, FSH is one of the hormones largely responsible for estrogen levels in the body. As estrogen levels decline as we age, FSH levels rise, reaching peak levels in menopause. Too much or too little can lead to infertility and menstrual difficulties.

LH (luteinizing hormone), like FSH, is produced in the pituitary gland and stimulates the ovaries to produce estrogen. A surge in LH triggers ovulation, the release of an egg from an ovarian follicle, in order to kick-start the fertile period of your cycle, and if fertilization occurs, LH pumps up to promote the production of progesterone to sustain the pregnancy. Just as with FSH, as estrogen levels decline as we age, LH levels rise, reaching peak levels in menopause. Too much or too little contributes to infertility.

What Reproductive Hormones Do During Fertility

Once puberty begins, a woman's reproductive system shifts into its baby-making role, trying at all costs to get an egg released, fertilized, and implanted. Knowing how your hormones ebb, flow, and work together during this roughly twenty-eight-day cycle will help you understand what's going on when your cycle starts to wind down during perimenopause and menopause. If you are still in perimenopause, I recommend tracking your menstrual cycle so that you can anticipate the changes in your cycle as you get closer to menopause.

Phase I: Menstruation (Days 1–7)

Day 1 of your cycle is always the first day of bleeding. Estrogen, progesterone, LH, and FSH are at their lowest levels. The progesterone dive causes the breakdown and shedding of the uterine lining—your period.

Phase II: Follicular Phase (Days 1–13)

This phase also starts on day one, but it extends for about a week after you've stopped bleeding. FSH, LH, estrogen, progesterone, and testosterone all gradually increase.

After the first few days of your period, the pituitary gland starts pumping out FSH to stimulate the follicles to mature and release more and more estrogen.

Rising estrogen tells your uterus to thicken the endometrial lining to create a cushy, nurturing home for a fertilized egg to implant.

Once estrogen levels max out, the pituitary gland turns down the FSH and amps up LH, the hormone primarily responsible for ovulation. Rising LH means rising testosterone, supporting follicular development and giving you your sexy mojo back just in time for ovulation.

Phase III: Ovulation (Day 14)

A single day with a sole purpose: time to make a baby! Ovulation is the main event of your menstrual cycle. Your body is ripe and juicy, feeling all the urges to get this egg fertilized.

Estrogen levels plummet just before LH surges, signaling the mature egg to burst from its follicle into the fallopian tube and down into the uterus. The egg has only a twenty-four-hour window to be fertilized or it will disintegrate. It's a short window, but a miraculous one!

Phase IV: Luteal Phase (Days 15–28)

Once ovulation occurs, the left-behind follicle transforms into something called a corpus luteum and begins to produce progesterone and estrogen. As these rise, FSH and LH drop. If ovulation doesn't occur, progesterone cannot be produced in the luteal phase, leading to low progesterone levels.

If the egg is fertilized, progesterone from the corpus luteum supports the early pregnancy. As your body creates a safe haven for baby, progesterone continues to rapidly increase. In the second trimester, the placenta takes over production of this hormone.

If the egg is not fertilized, the corpus luteum starts to break down, causing the drop in estrogen and progesterone levels that results in the shedding of your uterine lining. And the cycle begins all over again in the body's quest to reproduce.

What Reproductive Hormones Do During Perimenopause

Your body moves through this cycle, resetting and restoring each month for about twenty-five to thirty years when things eventually start to slow down. As we reach our mid thirties to early forties, the number and quality of our follicles diminish and they are less likely to release an egg; ironically, your body is more likely to release multiple eggs in a last-ditch effort to secure pregnancy, making multiples more common in women over age thirty-five. Erratic ovulation causes a few significant changes:

- Periods become irregular with cycle length and cycle flow varying from month to month. In your mid to late forties, you may lose your period for several months before it jumps back into action, and bleeding can go from lighter than normal to extremely heavy and back again.
- Estrogen levels become unpredictable and fluctuate rapidly, dropping precipitously and then spiking higher than normal.
- FSH and LH levels rise as the pituitary gland prods the ovaries to work harder and produce more estrogen in a last-ditch effort to restore balance for reproduction.
- Progesterone drops. Fewer ovulations means fewer opportunities for the corpus luteum to form and release this important hormone during the luteal phase of the cycle.
- Testosterone continues its anticipated age-related decline.

What Reproductive Hormones Do During Menopause

When your period has ceased for one year and you have officially entered menopause (yay!), your reproductive hormones have leveled out and your body gets off the monthly hormonal roller coaster. If you have had perimenopausal symptoms, this may allow them to decline or disappear.

- Estrogen, progesterone, and testosterone have decreased significantly and reached what we call their menopausal low. The ovaries are no longer producing them, and now the adrenal glands are tasked with producing enough to meet the body's needs.
- FSH and LH remain high.

Estrogen Dominance

Modern medicine leads us to believe that all of our perimenopause symptoms are caused by an estrogen deficiency resulting from ovarian decline and failure and that we should run out and get hormone therapy to raise estrogen. Listen to me now: The root of our symptoms in perimenopause isn't too little estrogen; it's too much.

Synthetic estrogens in the environment, cleaning, and personal care products contribute to a state known as estrogen dominance, when the body has too much estrogen and not enough progesterone to balance it out. It takes time for these extra estrogens to build up in your system, which is why far more women suffer from the effects of estrogen dominance during the transition to menopause. Excess estrogen has been piling up in our systems for years. Adding to our estrogen dominance is the fact that progesterone is the first hormone to decline during our forties. Women in menopause can have estrogen dominance, too. Even though estrogen levels do fall significantly after a woman's last period, it's the relationship between estrogen and progesterone that matters, not the individual level of each one. You can be low in estrogen but still have too much relative to progesterone.

Estrogen dominance is a near epidemic in my practice. Some women can suffer from the symptoms of estrogen dominance for ten to fifteen years, beginning as early as age thirty-five. I had estrogen dominance at the age of thirty-six, and it had a massive impact on my energy levels due to a lack of sleep most nights of the week. If left untreated, estrogen dominance can cause more serious concerns, such as fibroids, ovarian cysts, endometriosis, breast and uterine cancer, autoimmune diseases, and increased blood clotting.

Perimenopause is prime time for women to experience estrogen dominance, as the buildup of synthetic estrogens is overburdening our body and progesterone is on the decline. But these aren't the only causes. Why else could estrogen and progesterone deregulate? Here are just a few reasons:

- Too much stress taxes your adrenal glands, compromising their ability to produce progesterone.
- Excess body fat absorbs and stores estrogen, increasing estrogen levels.
- A sluggish liver is unable to remove excess estrogen.
- Birth control pills and hormone therapy containing synthetic or bioidentical estrogen can add fuel to the fire by piling on additional estrogen.

Estrogen dominance is not inevitable because of the changes to our reproductive hormones as we move through perimenopause and menopause. With awareness and proper lifestyle changes, we can get estrogen dominance under control.

Dismantling the Myth That You Must Be on Hormone Replacement Therapy (HRT) to Manage Menopause

The only reason you should be on hormone replacement therapy (HRT) is if you and your functional practitioner have discussed all of your symptoms, weighed all of your options, considered your risk factors and personal preferences, and determined it is right for you. You do not *need* to be on HRT. It is not required for good health, including strong bones, a healthy heart, or a sharp mind. Menopause is not a disease. Your body is not deficient and in need of an estrogen supplement to "fix" it. You can balance hormones *without* hormones!

HRT generally uses synthetic hormones to spot-treat your troublesome symptoms in hopes that you find some relief, much like an over-the-counter drug. The problem is that it masks symptoms and often creates its own set of new symptoms, just like it did for my mom. Before you resort to HRT, you need to be sure that your root causes are handled while firming up your foundation with solid nutrition and self-care techniques to support your gut and liver, and lower stress. Flooding your body with synthetic estrogen or slathering on progesterone cream isn't a good long-term solution if your cortisol levels are constantly elevated due to stress, your insulin fluctuates wildly because of poor diet, and your liver is working overtime to clear toxins. I view HRT as a last resort for short-term relief.

While we're at it, let's talk about bioidentical hormones, too. Some say they are a natural and safer option for hormone replacement. My answer? Yes and no. The word "natural" can be very misleading because every hormone used in hormone therapy, whether synthetic or bioidentical, is created in a lab. The difference is that synthetic hormones try to mimic the natural hormones your body produces, but have a slightly different chemical structure that is different from what our bodies create. Bioidentical hormones are still drugs, but they are made from phytoestrogens that are chemically identical to the ones produced by the human body. Made from yams and soy in the laboratory, bioidentical hormones have yielded some promising results and are considered breast, brain, and heart protective. The concern is that they aren't always regulated and researched well enough yet to be sure of their long-term consistency. When it comes to using bioidentical hormones for symptom management, I recommend trusting your intuition and always consider using natural solutions and lifestyle recommendations first.

If your symptoms persist, it's worth taking that first step on the road to using bioidentical hormones and evaluating your risk factors and medical history, including family history, so that you can create a clear picture of your health needs and goals. It's always important to take into account the whole body before introducing natural bioidentical hormones. While they can be very helpful in some instances, they may not fully address all of your symptoms on their own.

But Wait, There's More!

As you can see, there's a lot going on with your reproductive hormones, especially during perimenopause. But no matter what you may have been told, declining ovarian function and progesterone plus fluctuating estrogen levels are not the only reason you're feeling symptoms. Remember that grand symphony of hormones?

There are several other major hormones involved in how your body functions and how you feel, including cortisol, insulin, and thyroid hormones, just to name a few. If these hormones are out of whack—and trust me, most of the time they are—you will struggle. To feel like Superwoman again, we need to restore these hormones to balance and address the root causes (stress! toxins!) driving them to dysregulate in the first place.

Chapter 2

More Hormones That Matter During Menopause

We've been led to believe that lower estrogen levels are the reason for all of our peri/menopausal symptoms, but now we know there are many hormone players involved. Increasingly out-of-sync hormones, including insulin, cortisol, and thyroid hormones, exacerbate the hormonal changes you're already experiencing and increase your symptoms, from hot flashes and mood swings to belly fat and insomnia. But hormones don't become imbalanced on their own. There is always an underlying reason, a root cause, driving your hormones to work improperly. I have spent years getting to the bottom of what causes hormonal chaos because I saw women suffering, my mom suffered, and I began to suffer as well.

What I found is this: When we balance the hormones and treat the root causes that can compromise our gut and liver function, ramp up our stress, ruin our blood sugar balance, and wreck our thyroid, we eliminate many symptoms associated with peri/menopause and allow our bodies to function at optimal levels. Instead of applying a prescription Band-Aid for each individual symptom, we get to the root of the problem, the foundation of your structure, and work from the ground up.

The Role of Cortisol: When Stress Is a Root Cause of Hormonal Imbalance

Cortisol is your body's main stress hormone and is naturally produced in response to perceived stress, telling you to either fight the danger, flee for preservation, or freeze. But cortisol does a lot more than that, helping regulate blood sugar levels, reduce inflammation, and control your circadian rhythm, the twenty-four-hour internal clock that influences many bodily functions, including when you sleep and wake. It's a powerhouse hormone, and when it's in balance, it's a great friend to have. When it's out of balance, it is the source of the majority of hormone-related issues, especially perimenopause and menopause symptoms.

The production and release of cortisol is controlled by the hypothalamus, pituitary gland, and adrenals, a trio of glands often referred to as the HPA axis. It goes like this: When we encounter a stressor or perceived stressor, the hypothalamus, the brain's communications center, releases CRH (corticotropin-releasing hormone) to tell the pituitary gland that there's a potential threat. The pituitary gland, the body's master control gland in charge of telling all of the endocrine glands what to do, responds by instructing the adrenal glands to kick into action via ACTH (adrenocorticotropic hormone). The adrenals respond by producing cortisol to raise our blood sugar levels so we have enough fuel for the coming confrontation and suppress all nonessential systems. Digestion and reproduction take a back seat to improve our chances for survival.

Once the threat has passed and we perceive that the stressor has been eliminated, the body triggers a negative feedback loop from the adrenals to the pituitary to the hypothalamus to slow the secretion of CRH and ACTH. This returns cortisol levels to normal and resets the stress response system. All good!

The problem is, many of us don't return to balance, instead operating in chronic stress mode brought on by just about everything in day-to-day modern life: social media, work, never-ending to-do lists, environmental pollutants, inconsistent sleep schedules, and poor nutrition. Our HPA axis is constantly "on," and the flood of cortisol keeps the system in overdrive until it simply can't keep up. That's when we land in what's known as HPA axis dysfunction and total hormonal havoc—estrogen dominance, thyroid dysfunction, increased belly fat, PMS and heavy and painful periods, moodiness, sugar and carb cravings, and sleep troubles, to name a few! In other words, if your body is swamped with excess levels of cortisol and your HPA axis is sputtering, you'll feel it *everywhere*.

Two types of stress are usually at the root of a cortisol imbalance: perceived chronic stress and trauma.

Perceived Chronic Stress

One of the most fascinating things about stress is how individual it is. It's tough to objectively measure stress because no two people experience the same situation in exactly the same way. A tense meeting at work could raise your stress levels through the roof, while it doesn't faze me in the least. But a fight with my husband? Now, that gets my heart racing and cortisol soaring! To each her own!

Because stress is so subjective, we often measure it as "perceived stress," your perception of and thoughts and feelings about the amount of stress you are under and your ability to cope with it. It should come as no surprise that those who see their stress as overwhelming and sky-high are at greater risk for depression, heart disease, immune issues, infectious diseases, and premature aging.

By the time you feel chronically swamped by stress and helpless to cope with it, the more difficult it is to recover from the metabolic damage. As I discovered more than ten years ago, stress can be addictive, and unknowingly, your body gets used to the rush. Feeling stressed can easily become our new normal. That's why stress is the root cause rather than the result of most symptoms and conditions. Even small amounts of stress experienced on a daily basis can create a situation in which your body slips into hormonal imbalance.

You're going to be hearing a lot about stress throughout this book, because getting your perceived stress under control is essential for getting your hormone levels back on track and alleviating your menopause symptoms.

Trauma

When I was diagnosed with Hashimoto's back in 2018, I had a deep knowledge that my past unresolved trauma played a big role. Instead of addressing my trauma, I distracted myself with work and prided myself at being a high achiever. Because I used my work as a distraction, my trauma festered, and finally my body couldn't handle the stress, exhaustion, and deep-seated anger I had run from for many years. My autoimmunity was a clear sign to me that it was time for me to do some deeper healing work.

It's important to understand that what one's body perceives as traumatic can vary widely. You may be dealing with unresolved shock from traumatic events that you don't even realize, and PTSD doesn't just happen to war veterans. Witnessing, experiencing, or even empathetically responding to a traumatic event affects you at your core even if symptoms may not develop until later in life. Even a similar event or experience could trigger your stress response and revive memories that had been buried in your subconscious for years.

What I encourage you to do is to sit down and create a Health-Life Timeline. Start at the beginning with what kind of birthing experience your mother had and mark down every illness as well as major or minor events in your life. Any shocking or distressing event has the potential to impact our physical and emotional health in both the short and the long term: parental neglect, abuse, divorce, an accident, sexual assault, or natural disaster. Even something as seemingly innocuous as a childhood illness or a fender-bender should not be discounted as unimportant. Anything that pops into your mind may be valid, so take time and care when constructing your timeline. Don't be surprised if more and more events come to mind that may have relevance once you see where your health issues pop up in relation to the events.

You may not think that events from years ago, maybe even decades, still have the power to impact your health. You may not even remember the trauma clearly or at all. But the body remembers. To journey with more ease and grace through menopause, you must address and heal past trauma. I know that's easy to say and hard to do but I want you to know that there is a lot of good news around treating trauma and many effective ways to ease its impact.

Resources for Supporting Trauma

EFT, or Emotional Freedom Techniques, is a therapeutic psychological technique that utilizes a series of tapping with affirmative mantras to help the body release pent-up negativity in the moment.

Acupuncture stimulates points in the body using very thin needles that penetrate the skin, and should only be performed by a trained professional. Often, the process can relieve both pain and the stored emotional stress of traumatic experiences.

EMDR, or Eye Movement Desensitization and Reprocessing, is a psychotherapy technique using interactions between you and a trained professional to relieve the effects of psychological stress by triggering or reliving previous trauma while directing your eye movements. Studies have shown it to be greatly successful in breaking associations and triggers brought on by circumstances to alleviate symptoms.

Essential oils can powerfully support the body in releasing emotional trauma stored in the body through therapeutic massage.

Counseling allows you to talk through more intense issues with an uninvolved third party who can objectively guide you through the healing techniques best for your body, mind, and soul.

The Role of Insulin: When Dysregulated Blood Sugar Is a Root Cause of Hormonal Balance

Insulin is the hormone—produced by the pancreas—that allows your body to use blood sugar (glucose) for energy and keep blood sugar levels balanced. Whether or not you are diabetic or prediabetic, you should pay attention to insulin. It's even more important to do so in perimenopause and menopause, as the age-related changes our bodies are experiencing make it easier for this hormone to become imbalanced.

When you eat any type of carbohydrate, your body breaks it down into glucose, or blood sugar. As your blood sugar rises, insulin is released to carry the glucose from your bloodstream into cells throughout your body that need it for energy and return blood sugar levels to normal. When we eat too many carbs, generating more blood sugar than our cells need, the body converts glucose to glycogen and stores it in the liver or as fat. If we consistently eat too many carbs, continuously flooding the body with blood sugar and insulin, our cells lose their sensitivity to insulin and no longer respond to it. This is insulin resistance. And it's incredibly common, impacting one in three Americans—including half of those age sixty and older.

Now our blood sugar stays high and our insulin is high as the pancreas keeps pumping it out in a frantic bid to move glucose into cells. But those cells aren't listening! The blood sugar circulating in your body gets dumped into fat cells, especially around your middle, and your cells still crave fuel. You eat and eat, but stay hungry, not to mention tired and brain foggy. The pounds pack on while other hormones and bodily systems are thrown off-kilter.

Over time, your pancreas gets worn out from working so hard, and your risk for type 2 diabetes, heart attacks, strokes, and cancer increases. Elevated insulin and insulin resistance is no joke in perimenopause and menopause, especially with the drop in estrogen and progesterone. Now is the time to stabilize your levels, restore your insulin sensitivity, and put these symptoms in the rearview.

A poor diet is often the source of blood sugar and insulin imbalance. Cutting out processed foods and sugars and eating an organic plant-based whole food diet high in fiber and grass-fed animal protein will get you off the roller coaster. It supports balanced blood sugar while promoting restful sleep, a healthy weight, and a better, more stable mood.

The Role of Your Liver: When a Sluggish Liver Is a Root Cause of Hormonal Imbalance

More than 500 vital functions rely on the liver, the largest organ of the body, so trust me when I say you don't want your liver doing a second-rate job! It produces bile that aids your small intestine in breaking down fats, and it reduces carbs, protein, fats, vitamins, minerals, and other essential nutrients into basic compounds your body can use to stay strong.

Detoxification is the main job of your amazing liver. It works hard to detox your body of harmful substances each and every day. What you may not know is that those substances aren't just chemicals and toxins; they include excess and used-up hormones that need to be removed from circulation. A sluggish liver will slow down your body's natural filtration process, leading to an overload of harmful substances in the body and hormonal imbalance, especially estrogen. A healthy liver will detox the body of estrogen that has done its job, breaking it down and excreting it, but when the liver is overworked, the partially broken-down estrogen will spill back into our system, leading to estrogen dominance and all of the issues and risks associated with that condition.

Endocrine Disruptors (EDs) or Endocrine-Disrupting Chemicals, Including Heavy Metals

Supporting your liver by making sure it gets all of the nutrients it needs and reducing your exposure to damaging environmental toxins may be the missing link in your hormone health, especially during perimenopause and menopause. Endocrine disruptors (EDs), a specific type of widespread toxin, are a common culprit for an over-burdened liver and widespread hormonal imbalance. Found in many personal care products (including soaps, toothpastes, and cosmetics), plastics and food storage, cleaning products, and even nonstick cook-ware (among many other sources).

EDs are a dangerous group of chemicals because they pack a dou-ble wallop. First, they put a tremendous burden on our liver, forcing it to work extra hard to clear them from our body. Overwhelmed by toxins, the liver has a tough time clearing them, meaning many of them end up right back in our bloodstream. And a now-sluggish liver is spending all its energy trying to clear EDs instead of doing its other 500 (literally!) critical functions. No wonder the symptoms of toxic overload and a struggling liver are so wide-ranging!

The second wallop—hormone imbalance—is baked right into their name. As endocrine disruptors, these chemicals interfere with your endocrine system, where hormones are produced and function. Some block and bind hormone receptors, preventing natural hormones from doing their job, while others impact how hormones are made, broken down, or stored. Another kind mimics naturally occurring hormones and prevents the natural hormones your body makes from entering your cells. For example, xenoestrogens are a type of ED that imper-sonates estrogen. The most important thing to understand is that even the smallest amount can have a very big impact on your body, which is why EDs are often measured in parts per *trillion,* or ppt, and they are very stable, meaning they are difficult to purge from your bodily systems.

In addition to the chemical EDs, we also need to be concerned with the amount of heavy metals present in our lives, as these also strain our liver and disrupt our hormones. Not only can they leach into the water, soil, and air supply through agricultural and industrial waste, but they are most definitely lurking in your home, in your refrigerator, on your body, and even in the metal fillings in your teeth. Most of us know to avoid lead in paint, arsenic in cigarette smoke, and mercury in tuna, but lots of heavy metals get into our systems, one tiny bit at a time: a little mercury in your go-to lip gloss, a bit of aluminum in your favorite antiperspirant, a smidge of cadmium and nickel as you brush on the whitening toothpaste, and a trace of lead chipping off with your nail polish. Yikes! And they are extremely difficult to break down and detox out of your body.

While it's impossible to completely avoid EDs and heavy metals, there are ways to limit your exposure and minimize their impact. Switching to natural or DIY versions of beauty and personal care products as well as cleaning supplies, filtering your water with a reverse osmosis filter, and being sure you know where and how your food is grown can be the first steps toward getting control back. Reducing your toxic load will have a huge impact on restoring the natural ebb and flow of your hormones.

The Role of Your Digestive Issues: When Gut Issues Are a Root Cause of Hormonal Imbalance

Guess what symptom most women with hormonal imbalance all have in common? Yup, digestive distress. But it is more than just a bit of bloating passed off as PMS symptoms. There is a deeper force at work here that scientists understand more and more each day. The depth of how our gut affects our overall systemic health continues to astound me, which is why I always suggest that women make over their nutrition and begin to heal their gut immediately when they come to me. What I have often found is that women are caught in an intestinal catch-22 situation: They go to the doctor with gut issues, get diagnosed with IBS or another issue, begin taking prescriptions that mess with their hormones, stress themselves out about it, and guess what happens when your body gets stressed and cortisol ramps up? It shuts your digestive system down. So, back to the doctor you go, and the cycle perpetuates from medicine to medicine, not really getting to the bottom of your issue. Sound familiar?

Like your liver, your gut plays a pivotal role in your total hormonal health. So much so that some scientists consider the microbiome, the trillions of microbes living inside your intestines, an endocrine organ. The gut microbiome not only produces over two dozen hormones but acts as a conductor, directing the other endocrine glands to make and release hormones. The gut microbiome influences nearly every hormone in your body, including estrogen, cortisol, and thyroid hormones.

Its impact on estrogen can't be underestimated. When the liver is done breaking down and deactivating estrogen, it sends it to your intestines, where a group of bacteria, the estrobolome, goes to work reducing it even further until it's eventually excreted in your stool. If too many bad bacteria have taken over your microbiome and the good bacteria in the estrobolome can't do their job, the deactivated estrogen isn't fully metabolized and eliminated, but is sent back into your bloodstream—a perfect storm for estrogen dominance.

Leaky Gut and Gut Dysbiosis

When your gut is healthy, your hormones are in harmony. But when your gut ain't happy, ain't nobody happy! Get ready for a parade of issues, from digestive distress (constipation, gas, bloating, heartburn, diarrhea, and stomach pains) to mood swings and sleep problems.

Leaky gut and gut dysbiosis are likely at the root of your digestive distress and hormone woes.

Leaky gut occurs when the gut lining becomes permeable, meaning things can slip through, allowing bacteria, food particles, and other toxins to "leak" into the body and the bloodstream. When this happens, the immune system launches an attack to fight these invaders and inflammation skyrockets, causing IBS, food allergies and sensitivities, skin issues, and autoimmune diseases like hypothyroidism or rheumatoid arthritis. And, of course, hormone imbalance.

Gut dysbiosis refers to an unhealthy microbiome, when the bad bacteria and microbes begin to outnumber the beneficial ones that usually keep your microbiome in check. Gut dysbiosis negatively impacts many systems, but it directly influences your estrogen levels by harming the estrobolome.

Both issues can lead to digestive distress—constipation or diarrhea, a combination of both, bloating, cramping, and general discomfort—as well as prevent the adequate absorption of vitamins, minerals, and antioxidants necessary to support your hormonal production. You may be taking supplements and medications to help support your overall health, but your broken digestive system is making it difficult to absorb them!

Stress (especially stress!), a diet high in processed and inflammatory foods, gut infections, and toxins are a few of the main drivers of leaky gut and gut dysbiosis.

Reclaiming your digestive health by addressing leaky gut and gut dysbiosis is essential for reclaiming your hormonal health.

Nutrient Deficiencies

It's pretty simple: If you're stressed and your gut is in bad shape, your body isn't getting the nutrients it needs for hormone production and cellular energy, and it won't function optimally. The typical American diet of highly processed foods loaded with added sugar, refined flours, and industrial seed oils not only does serious damage to your intestinal lining and microbiome but provides empty calories with zero nutrients. Sadly, more than half the calories Americans consume come from these nutrient-depleted, ultra-processed foods with predictable results.

Eating real food—clean protein, healthy fats, and fiber as lots of organic fruits and veggies—is the answer to heal your gut and get most of the nutrients, vitamins, and minerals you need. That said, even with a super clean, plant-based, fiber-filled, whole food diet, it's difficult to get *all* of the nutrients we need, especially magnesium, vitamin D, zinc, and the B-complex vitamins. High-quality supplements are the most efficient way to fill in the nutrient gaps. While your diet should provide the majority of your dietary needs, sometimes our genetic makeup prevents proper metabolization or methylation of the nutrients that we need. In that case, supplementation is absolutely necessary.

In most cases, to assess your nutrient levels, simple blood panels can be taken, so be sure to advocate for yourself and see if a nutrient deficiency could be at the root of your symptoms. Results don't need to be flagged as low for you to be concerned, either. Each individual needs their own healthy levels of nutrients, so aim for somewhere in the middle of the acceptable levels. If you are near the low end, you might want to revisit your nutrition. And if you are flagged as low, it may take some targeted supplementation over time to increase those levels plus some gut TLC to make sure you actually absorb them.

The Role of the Thyroid: When Poor Function Is a Root Cause of Hormonal Imbalance

Many women in perimenopause and menopause are struggling with low thyroid function, or hypothyroidism. Between ages thirty-five and sixty-five, about 13 percent of women will have an underactive thyroid, rising to 20 percent among those over sixty-five. The numbers are probably much higher, though, as many women are undiagnosed. I know because I fell into the undiagnosed category for more than two years, and so did many of the women I have helped. Standard tests are inadequate (see The Importance of Testing on page 284 for testing recommendations) and the signs are often dismissed or ignored because they are so similar to the symptoms of perimenopause: brain fog, hot flashes, stubborn weight gain, fatigue, irritability, low libido, insomnia, hair loss, and dry skin. These are so wide-ranging because your thyroid does a lot of heavy lifting within your body.

A butterfly-shaped gland in the front of your neck, the thyroid is responsible for regulating hundreds of functions, from metabolism to body temperature. In addition, every human cell has thyroid hormone receptors. Your entire body, including your brain, muscles, heart, intestines, and immune system, depends on adequate thyroid hormones to be at their best. The main thyroid hormones are:

TSH (thyroid-stimulating hormone) is produced in the pituitary gland and stimulates the production of T4 (thyroxine) and T3 (triiodothyronine).

T3 (triiodothyronine) is the playmaker in the thyroid hormone squad, directly affecting nearly every physiological process in your body, including body temperature, cholesterol, energy, heart rate, memory, menstrual cycle, muscle strength, weight, and more. The liver converts it from T4 and other tissues.

Thyroxine (T4) is your main thyroid hormone directly secreted by the thyroid gland into the bloodstream in inactive form and functions as a storage component for T3. It must be converted to T3 by the liver and kidneys in order to be used by the body. Its levels trigger the production or cessation of TSH by the pituitary gland.

If your thyroid is functioning optimally, it is able to easily maintain a stable balance of T3 and T4. When levels drop, the pituitary releases TSH to trigger the thyroid to produce T4, which converts to T3. As soon as T3 and T4 are back to normal levels, TSH production slows and everything holds steady. When it's not functioning optimally, an underproduction of these hormones will slow down the body's metabolism, causing hypothyroidism. (An excess will speed up metabolism, resulting in hyperthyroidism.)

Low thyroid function can have several causes:

- Our old friend estrogen dominance can reduce the availability of thyroid hormones for use in the cells.
- Stress can screw up these hormones in so many ways! It slows thyroid function, fatigues the pituitary gland so it doesn't make enough TSH, prevents cells from being able to use thyroid hormones because of increased inflammation, and—well, you get the idea.
- An autoimmune disease in which the immune system "targets" the thyroid. The most common is Hashimoto's thyroiditis.
- Too little or too much iodine in your diet can negatively impact the production of thyroid hormone. In most cases, it's too much iodine.
- Toxins can directly damage the thyroid gland, making it less responsive to TSH.

If you were to look at side-by-side lists of symptoms of hypothyroidism and hyperthyroidism, and perimenopause and menopause, you would be amazed at the parallels. Indeed, it's paramount that we make sure this gland is in tip-top condition and do all we can to support it.

Quiz: What Is Causing Perimenopause and Menopause Hormonal Imbalances?

I have created a comprehensive Perimenopause and Menopause Hormone Quiz, which is designed to help you determine the root causes of your perimenopause or menopause symptoms so that you can best use this book. Once you know the root causes, you can focus on implementing targeted whole food nutrition, supplementation, essential oils, and self-care protocols to get your body back on track. Before continuing with Part II of this book, go to www.drmariza.com/hormonequiz and take the quiz.

Finding Hormone Balance

How can you even begin to address the multiple hormonal imbalances causing you grief? What if you think you have several root causes—or all of them—at the core of the problem? Don't freak out. You are in the right place. I have been there and had my own panic session when I was researching root causes and realized that I had several of my own! It became my mission to find a starting place for every woman. Here it is: a hormone-balancing trifecta to reset your gut, liver, and stress.

Targeting these top-line problem areas with foundational lifestyle changes gets at the most common and damaging root causes to restore your energy and radiance and kick those perimenopause and meno-pause symptoms to the curb. No matter what your unique root causes turn out to be, you will benefit from healing your gut, detoxifying your liver, and lowering your stress. We're going to go about it with healing foods, movement, stress reduction, supplementation, and perhaps the most powerful tool in any healing toolbox: essential oils.

Chapter 3

Restore Your Radiance— Using Essential Oils to Support Your Hormonal Balance

I honestly cannot imagine my life without the daily usage of essential oils. The many chemical constituents in essential oils impact your body at the cellular level to both address the symptoms for immediate relief while simultaneously supporting the body's ability to heal from within. Just one drop can massively impact your emotional and physical well-being and alleviate your perimenopausal or menopausal symptoms. Of course, everyone responds to essential oils differently, so it is very important to be aware of how you feel after using each kind of oil.

Unlike many over-the-counter and prescribed remedies, essential oils can be used as often as you like. Imagine not waiting forty minutes for pain relief to cycle throughout your entire system! Essential oils also don't mask symptoms like many of the over-the-counter meds do, but instead provide sustained relief. They support your body's own healing miracles from the inside out and the outside in. This is true functional healing. While using plants to support your body's natural processes is a centuries-old practice, essential oil popularity has skyrocketed in the last ten years. Oils are popping up everywhere, but there is no central agency that approves essential oils for public usage. And many appear on the market with only basic instructions for use. It's therefore that much more important that you understand how, why, and when to use them properly.

Support with Essential Oils

In my time as a healthcare practitioner, I have researched, studied, and recommended a variety of functional protocols to my patients, none of which created instant wins like essential oils.

The immediate support that they offer is unparalleled, which is why they've been used for hundreds of years for their potency and power. I'll never forget when I learned that inhaling Peppermint was enough to overcome my crazy chocolate craving I had at three p.m. one afternoon. Peppermint has been a go-to oil for cravings ever since. What else works like that? But before we get into what essential oils *can* do, let me take a minute to explain what they *can't* do.

False Expectations for Essential Oils

Even though essential oils exhibit specialized properties and are composed of hundreds of potent constituents, they are not hormones! They cannot mimic estrogen or progesterone. Essential oils can't become hormones. They can't produce hormones. They can't replace hormones. Nature just doesn't work that way.

But nature gave us these amazing gifts that *can* support our bodies in healing themselves and that affects our bodies in miraculous ways. In other words, you can *treat* hormones without hormones.

Essential oils aren't the solution here—they are the *support*. Use them as tools to get you to the end game: healthy hormonal balance. But they won't get you there if you neglect lifestyle choices that establish the foundation for your good health.

How Essential Oils Can Support Hormones Without Adding Hormones

From my first whiff of Wild Orange, I was hooked on the healing power of essential oils, but the biochemist in me wouldn't let me dive in without first knowing all of the details. I studied book after book on essential oils and pored over hundreds of peer-reviewed articles. Soon I learned that they could be used to make over many aspects of our lives. Everything from your cleaning cabinet to your medicine cabinet can be revived with natural alternatives! And even better than that, their chemical constituents support your body on a cellular level, restoring your homeostasis to prevent and alleviate peri/menopausal symptoms.

Essential oils are adaptogenic, meaning they are made from plant substances known as adaptogens that help our bodies adapt to the internal and external environmental factors causing stress in our lives. They are able to support the body systemically through cellular support for hormone balance, our immune system, and overall homeostasis. They can calm, uplift, ground, and/or energize, with quick and effective results. As you will learn in this chapter, simply inhaling an essential oil immediately triggers the limbic system of the brain and prompts your body into supportive and healing action.

Choosing Essential Oils Wisely

I use only essential oils that have been specifically manufactured for therapeutic use and that meet scientific testing standards, and in the Resources section on page 357, I list those that I trust and use myself. Still, I think it's important to know that essential oils also come in food and perfume grades for use in a wide range of products you see in the market every day. At these lower grades, the oils are mostly just scenting products, masking the scents of the chemicals that give the product its cleaning or cosmetic power. But this kind of adulterated oil—those meant for food or perfume use—can do a lot of harm to your body and will not provide you with the healing results detailed in this book. Solvents and chemicals are often used to quicken the distillation process, and often "pure" oils are actually diluted versions that won't even begin to help you on your healing journey. If you react to a lesser-quality oil, you won't be able to tell if you're reacting to the essential oil or a poor production process that leaves junk behind. Yuck!!!

How do I assess quality? Well, I am particular! The companies that I trust set their own quality standards and strictly adhere to them. In addition to knowing these unique quality standards, I get answers to this list of necessaries, expecting a "yes" to each question (or at least the majority of them):

  Does the company clearly disclose where each essential oil is sourced?

  Are the plants harvested at peak times to ensure the highest-quality product?

  Are quality testing procedures utilized to ensure potency and purity?

  Does the company test for microbial properties?

  Are both gas chromatography and mass spectrometry tests done to ensure the highest quality? (Both must be used to verify the existence of correct compounds and the absence of harmful impurities in the final product.)

  Do partnerships exist between local growers and harvesters for a mutually beneficial relationship?

  Are the leaders trustworthy, using sound business practices?

If you are pressed for time and don't want to do this research yourself, check out the link I provide in the Resources section, but then also simply look at the bottle. Is it made of amber- or dark-colored glass to protect the essential oils from light? Is it tightly capped, upright, and fitted with an orifice reducer to prevent evaporation? (An orifice reducer is a plastic insert on the top of the bottle that seals the contents from air exposure and allows the oil to come out one drop at a time.) If the bottle doesn't look right, move on.

Once you get the essential oil home, you need to trust your own senses as you begin to use the oil. When you uncap the bottle, the smell should be prominent, crisp and clean, and balanced. Put a single drop of oil onto your fingertips and rub it into your skin to see if it leaves a residue. Watch it absorb into your skin, which should happen quickly with only a clean scent left behind. If the smell gives you a headache, doesn't absorb, causes a rash, leaves behind residue, or creates any other uneasy feeling, I would proceed with extreme caution or just stop using it altogether.

If your senses approve it, you still need to pay attention to the oil's potency. If you have to use more than one to two drops to achieve your desired results, it is probably a lesser-quality or diluted oil. Plus, if you are consistently using the oil and experiencing no benefits, then something is wrong. Or if you discover that over time your skin starts to react to it, discontinue use.

It is safer to purchase your essential oils from a trusted company that is transparent about its practices. The larger companies tend to have the resources to produce the high-grade essential oils that you desire to support your body in its healing miracles. I would buy only directly from the company's site, though some also stock their products in specialty and natural stores. As easy as online purchasing is, be sure to do your homework first. That said, I would not recommend ordering essential oils from a mass-market retailer like Amazon without first being sure that it is a certified product. Always check for opened bottles and broken seals on your bottles if you do opt to purchase nondirect online.

How to Effectively Use Essential Oils

Before beginning to implement essential oils as a part of your self-care healthcare plan, be sure to discuss them with your trusted healthcare provider or team, or an essential oil expert. Preexisting conditions, current prescription medications, and even natural supplementation could affect how the essential oils work for your unique body.

There are three main ways to use essential oils: aromatically, topically, and internally. Remember to check for the aromatic/topical/ internal usage on each individual oil, as each oil has different recommendations. Please know that the uses that I suggest in this book are acceptable for high-quality therapeutic-grade essential oils. If the bottle of oil in your hand is not labeled for the use I have suggested, then you probably need a higher-quality oil, as you will not achieve the expected results with one of lesser quality. And I need to say this just one more time: Your unique body chemistry will respond differently to both the individual oils and the protocols recommended in this book. It may take a little trial and error to figure out your preferred usage method and the most effective protocols for your body.

Aromatic Use

The easiest and fastest way to benefit from essential oils is breathing them in aromatically. Their volatile nature allows essential oils to quickly evaporate and pervade the area around you, directly influencing your mood, memory, emotions, and hormones.

After entering through the nose and lungs, the constituents of the essential oils stimulate the receptors in the brain's olfactory system. The mitral cells receive the output signals and carry them from the olfactory bulb to the limbic brain, the command center for a myriad of bodily functions including memory, sleep, emotional and hormonal regulation. But the essential oils reach other areas of the brain and body as well. Breathing in essential oil enables it to enter your bloodstream, where it takes a ride around the body, positively influencing and supporting areas in need. Excretion takes place through the kidneys, lungs, and pores, but not before powerfully affecting the endocrine system, home base for hormone production. The HPA axis can be directly supported with essential oils, and with the stressed-out world we live in, it needs all the support it can get!

The term "aromatic" includes direct and indirect inhalation as well as homemade steamers and several different methods of diffusion. Let's look at this in turn.

DIRECT INHALATION

This is pretty much what it sounds like: Simply smelling the oil directly from the bottle. For your first inhale of a new oil, crack the top and hold the bottle at arm's length away from your face, then slowly bring it toward your chin while inhaling. This should always be the first way to assess a new oil. Patch testing is the next step (see page 66) before moving on to the Palm Method. This involves putting a single drop of oil in your palm, rubbing your palms together, and then cupping them over your mouth and nose while inhaling deeply.

INDIRECT INHALATION

There are several different ways to indirectly inhale essential oils. You can place one to two drops on an object that allows for sustained aroma, such as a tissue or cotton ball, a piece of wood, or diffuser jewelry that includes felt, leather, or lava beads.

STEAMERS

Heating up water until it steams and then adding essential oils gives a lung-opening aromatic experience like no other. I love a good steamer when congestion clogs up my ability to breathe freely. I also love putting a few drops of oil on a cotton ball and putting it in my shower, so the steam can create my own therapeutic spa experience.

AROMATIC SPRAYS

Freshen up any room (I like a spritz in the shower), clothing, or bed-clothes by adding ten to fifteen drops of essential oil to a 2-ounce glass spray bottle and topping off with distilled water or witch hazel. Cap and shake to combine. Shake well before spraying.

DIFFUSERS

Diffusing is one of my favorite ways to use essential oils to support my mood, immunity, and energy levels. The most popular and standard type of diffuser is an ultrasonic cool-air diffuser, which utilizes distilled water, four to six drops of oil, and ultrasonic vibrations to create a fine airborne mist. It suspends the oils into the air for sustained release as you continue to breathe in the benefits. All of the diffuser recipes in this book were created for an ultrasonic cool-air diffuser, but be sure to use your manufacturer's guidelines for your specific machine. And be sure to clean it naturally using 1 part white vinegar with 2 parts water and letting it soak. It is also recommended that you diffuse for fifteen to thirty minutes at a time and then take a 45-to-60-minute break for your olfactory system; otherwise the effects of the oil may be diminished.

Note: Avoid using any product with a heating element that touches the oil, as it breaks down the chemical constituents and reduces effectiveness. Also avoid humidifiers and vaporizers, since their components (often plastic) were not manufactured for essential oils. High-quality essential oils are so powerful that they can break down plastics, causing toxins to leach out into the air and slowly destroying the machine.

Topical Use

Topical, or direct, application means simply applying the oils right where they are needed on the skin for a direct effect. Applying oils topically can be very effective and instantaneous—remember the power of one drop!

Once you have passed the aromatic test, topical usage can exponentially increase the benefits reaped from these single drops of high-quality essential oils. As the constituents travel through your body, they affect every area they pass, providing support to those that need it before being excreted. The powerful chemical constituents of essential oils quickly absorb into your skin, combine with its natural sebum, and directly enter the bloodstream for healing miracles!

NEAT VERSUS DILUTED

The potency of high-quality therapeutic essential oils requires special care when applying topically. For that reason, we use two terms when directing topical application: neat and diluted. **Neat** means direct application of oil to skin, while **Diluted** means adding a high-quality carrier oil to the essential oil (not water, which repels oil) before application. Let's look at the benefits and cautions of each method.

Neat application works for some people, but for those with more sensitive skin, it may not. There are certain oils such as Lavender and Frankincense that I always use neat on my skin, but I always recommend dilution to others until you know how your body responds. If you apply an oil neat and begin to experience a reaction, you should *always* dilute with a carrier oil.

Dilution enables more widespread absorption of the oil, lessening the pinpoint effect when you drop only onto a small area. It does not require a complicated process and can be easily accomplished once you find your preferred carrier oil(s) (see page 62 for a list). That said, you can experience a reaction to carrier oils, so be sure to test them first. Adverse dermal reactions can be irritating, and dilution can lessen the likelihood or intensity of a potential irritation. The lipophilic properties of essential oils enable them to easily combine with other natural oils and fatty substances, decreasing their potency. I love using raw organic cold-pressed unrefined coconut oil (solid form) and fractionated coconut oil (liquid form) for dilution in my rollerball bottle protocols, but other favorites include grapeseed, jojoba, and sweet almond oil. When preparing a dilution for your face, I highly recommend using jojoba since it most closely resembles the natural sebum of your skin. But the light scent and additional benefits of sweet almond oil and coconut oil make them my favorite for massage and everyday use.

WHERE DO I APPLY ESSENTIAL OILS?

While the recipes and protocols in this book will always contain recommended application techniques, I invite you to listen to your body and apply where they work the best for you. It may take a while to find your sweet spot for each oil, but once you do, I promise it will be life-changing! Knowing your body and trusting your gut provides a magic touch to your essential oil arsenal. For starters, though, there are three key things I always tell my patients:

#1 **Apply Where Needed:** A rule of thumb for essential oil application is to always apply the oil as close as possible to the area in need. For instance, is a hot flash threatening to cause embarrassing sweat pouring through your clothes? Apply some Peppermint on the back and front of your neck for a cooling focal point and instant relief. An important exception: If a tension headache causes halos in your eyesight, do not apply the oils directly to your eyelids. Instead, opt for your temples or your forehead. The oils will go where they are needed once applied.

#2 **Apply to Pulse Points:** Anywhere you can check your pulse provides an optimal application site for essential oils: behind your ears, on your neck, at your temples, on your wrists and ankles, and over your heart. Now, this doesn't mean you should apply oils to all of these spots at the same time. Experiment to find the one site or combination of sites that works the best for you.

#3 **Apply to FEW Spots** (Feet, Ears, Wrists): The skin on the bottom of your feet, your ears, and your wrists is thin, and the pores are large. Eastern medicine often recommends application to the bottoms of your feet, touted as the pipelines to the body for quick absorption and ultimate effect. Paired with reflexology, the application of appropriate pressure to specific points and areas on the feet, hands, or ears, strategic application by gentle massage of essential oils can power-fully support your system. Application to the ears and wrists provides a bonus aromatherapeutic benefit with quick absorption and delivery to the neediest areas of your body.

HOW DO I APPLY ESSENTIAL OILS?

You have several choices for how to apply essential oils: layered, through massage or compress, tented, or through a bath soak.

Layered: This approach means applying one oil at a time, one directly on top of the other, in a specific order for optimum benefits.

- Apply one oil first and give it a few seconds to absorb before applying the next.
- Repeat until all have been applied.

> **Tip:** Use a "driver" oil like Peppermint last to increase absorption of the other oils and/or apply a warm, wet compress using the water to repel the oils deeper into your skin.

Massage: This refers to using a carrier oil and your hands to work the oils into the skin. For therapeutic massage, add one to two drops of an essential oil to 1 teaspoon (5 ml) of carrier oil.

- Prep massage oil ahead by using 25 drops of essential oil to 1 teaspoon of carrier oil and store in an airtight glass jar or rollerball bottle.

> **Note:** For beginners, use slow, gentle strokes with light pressure with essential oils.

Compress: When you put a wet compress on top of an essential oil you have applied directly to the skin, you push the oils in deeper, using the water-repels-oil science.

- Use a warm compress for muscle stiffness or aches and pains.

- Use a cool compress for inflammation, swelling, spasms, or acute injuries.
- Warm creates more aromatherapeutic benefits, while cool can soothe away hot flashes.

Tented: This is more elaborate-sounding than it really is! You simply apply essential oils topically along your décolletage and then tuck your mouth and nose into your shirt and breathe deeply; for obvious reasons this method is also known as the "T-shirt tent."

- Be sure to alternate a few deep breaths inside the tent and then a few outside the tent.
- Repeat until you feel relief.
- This provides a double benefit of topical and aromatherapeutic effects.

> **Note:** Women with preexisting respiratory conditions should proceed with caution when using this technique. If any concerns arise, consult with a trusted health practitioner.

Bath Soak: Combining Epsom salts, warm bathwater, and essential oils makes for a toxin-releasing and muscle-relaxing experience.

- Add 2 cups of Epsom salts to warm bathwater, swirling to combine before adding 3 to 6 drops of essential oils.
- Epsom salts help the oils to disperse in the bathwater and absorb into your body (without them, the oils will just float on top of the water).
- Magnesium in the Epsom salts will relax your body and improve restful sleep.
- Soak for 20 minutes and then rinse off to wash the released toxins down the drain. Be sure to hydrate well both before and after your soak.

Internal Use

Despite the increasing science supporting the ingestion of essential oils, the essential oil community continues to debate the efficacy of this practice. I do not include internal usage recommendations in this book because there is no way to guarantee the quality of your essential oils. Many essential oils on the market are not safe to ingest. That said, I personally love to add essential oils to my smoothies and even to teas and my on-the-go glass-bottled water infusions, but I know my body and I know how these oils work to support my immune system and personal hormonal balance. My husband and I often use essential oils to spice up our cooking and add zing to desserts, but only those that are labeled as GRAS (generally recognized as safe) to ensure certification.

It is *not* recommended to take essential oils internally while pregnant or breastfeeding unless you have the guidance of a healthcare professional.

Synergistic Blends

While individual essential oils harness their own unique power, I will often recommend blends for the ultimate synergy of primary and secondary constituents. Years of research have led me to develop my own protocols and blends that thousands of women have successfully utilized to support their own bodies. I have carefully researched and incorporated the three categories of essential oils—calming/soothing, uplifting/energizing, and grounding/balancing—into synergistic blends that will support your body in incredible ways. In addition, I have personally used them myself and found great success in helping my body heal when used alongside the foundational lifestyle changes I detail in this book. The goal for you is to enjoy the experience while reaping the health benefits.

The method of use also varies from individual to individual, so be sure to give each oil and each blend an honest try. Our bodies need different things at different times, and results can come down to the specific places that you topically apply the oil or blend. Often layering the oils in a specific order will also produce a more powerful effect on your body. I recommend having fun with the discovery and working with the blends found in this book to find out the specific ways that they most effectively support your individual needs.

The Secret Weapon in Your Purse

I never leave home without essential oils in my purse and use them all day long to support my body, mood, and emotional well-being. Always on hand is my Instant Motivation Rollerball Blend (page 132), which combines the power of Peppermint, Rosemary, Wild Orange and Frankincense to give me a boost when I'm dragging or feeling unmotivated. I keep my oils safe in an essential oil case, basically a makeup clutch with elasticized loops inside to hold your favorite oils in place. (For where to get your own, see page 357 in Resources.)

Essential Oil Supplies

There's a steep learning curve when it comes to essential oil terminology that can be frustrating for a beginner, so here is a breakdown of the lingo for you! Plus, these basic supplies will equip you on your healing journey with essential oils.

Carrier Oils

Used in dilution, carrier oils are any neutral vegetable, nut, or seed oil that blends well with essential oils. Organic cold-pressed or expeller-pressed oils are the best to avoid any solvents or chemicals used in the refining process. Here are my favorites:

Organic Cold-Pressed Unrefined Coconut Oil

- Opaque white semisolid at room temperature with long shelf life
- Melts into a clear liquid when slightly warmed (even rubbing between your fingers will melt it!)
- Slight coconutty scent and complements most essential oil aromas

Organic Cold-Pressed Refined Coconut Oil

- Opaque white semisolid at room temperature with long shelf life
- Melts into a clear liquid when slightly warmed (even rubbing between your fingers will melt it!)
- Unscented

Fractionated Coconut Oil (FCO)

- Clear liquid at room temperature with long shelf life
- Perfect for basic dilution and easy usability, especially in a pump bottle
- Unscented

Jojoba Oil

- Clear golden liquid at room temperature with long shelf life
- Greaseless and easily absorbable; preferable for blends applied to the face
- Slightly nutty scent (unrefined version)

Sweet Almond Oil

- Clear pale yellow liquid at room temperature with short shelf life
- Rich in vitamins B and E and blends well with many oils
- Slightly nutty scent
- Avoid if you have a tree nut allergy

Grapeseed Oil

- Clear yellow to yellow-green liquid at room temperature with short shelf life
- Light oil great for massage blends
- Subtle sweet scent (made from the seeds of grapes)

Containers

All essential oils should come in tightly capped dark glass bottles (an exception is a rollerball, see below) and have an orifice reducer, dropper top, or rollerball to control the flow of oil.

Bottles

- 5-, 10-, and 15-milliliter bottles are standard sizes for high-quality therapeutic essential oils
- All should be tightly fitted with orifice reducers or dropper tops

Rollerball Bottles

- 5- and 10-milliliter slender bottles fitted with plastic or stainless steel rollerball tops
- Perfect for diluted blends and easy application
- May come in clear glass due to frequent usage
- Watch out for cloudy oil, meaning dead skin cells have infiltrated your oil and it's time to replace!

Personal Inhalers

- Small, torpedo-shaped plastic containers that fit snugly in the nostril
- Focused diffusion of specific essential oil blends
- Discreet and travel easily in your purse

Essential Oil Safety Recommendations

I love essential oils as fast-acting solutions because they are potent and effective at delivering relief to hormone-driven symptoms. Given their potency and strength, I want to provide you with some simple recommendations when using essential oil for everyday health concerns.

#1 Dilution

Starting with diluted oils will not decrease their efficacy, but it will decrease their potency. Dilution also enables a more widespread application on the body when you are focusing on a bigger area of concern. These potent little drops pack a punch of power, some more than others. And while most oils will not cause any sensation on the skin, there are hot and cool oils that leave a warming or tingly-cooling sensation after application. These oils should *always* be diluted before application. If they are not diluted, hot oils can irritate the skin and cooling oils can cross the line into an uncomfortable chilling sensation.

Hot oils include Cassia, Cinnamon, Cinnamon Bark, Clove, Thyme, Hyssop, and Oregano.

Cool oils include Camphor, Eucalyptus, Lemongrass, Ocotea, Peppermint, Spearmint, Thyme, and Wintergreen.

#2 Oil Repels Water

Way back in elementary school, we all learned the basic scientific principle that oil repels water, and vice versa. Oils will not wash off of your fingers with only water, and even soap may not do the trick. When essential oils need to be washed off, dilute first with a carrier oil and then add soap before adding water to the mix. If you have essential oil on your fingers and inadvertently touch a sensitive area of your body, such as your eyes, always dilute, dilute, dilute with a carrier oil. Even olive oil or vegetable oil will work in a pinch. That said, when you want to drive oils deeper into the skin, a warm compress has proven to be very effective in pushing the oils directly and deeply to the area that most needs support. I personally love this technique when I am applying Lavender and Frankincense to ease my neck tension at night.

#3 Patch Testing

Patch testing is the best way to check for any sensitivities or reactions to essential oils. It is an easy process. Simply add one drop of essential oil to 1 teaspoon of carrier oil and rub on a small area of your body. Each time you try a new essential oil, patch-test it on a small area of your skin—I recommend the best place to start is the bottoms of the feet—and wait twenty-four hours. Then move on to the area where you intend to apply the oil for maximum benefit. If you do have a reaction to the essential oil, remember *not* to wash it off with water, because the water will only push the oil in deeper. Dilute the area with more carrier oil over the next few hours until the area of irritation is gone, and be sure to contact your healthcare provider if you have any lingering concerns over the reaction.

#4 Reactions Versus Allergies/Sensitivities

In order for an essential oil to give you an adverse reaction—a rash, for instance—the plant protein must be present in the oil. Most proteins are actually removed during the oil distillation process. Still, reactions do sometimes happen, almost always because you have not diluted the essential oil enough. If there is a skin reaction, be sure to dilute with more carrier oil instead of washing it off with water. If you are allergic to a certain plant or flower or spice, proceed with using the essential oil with caution, because you may have a reaction from the aroma alone even if you don't touch the essential oil. And always contact your trusted healthcare provider with any concerns.

#5 Phototoxicity/Photosensitivity

An oil is categorized as phototoxic if it contains a primary constituent that reacts with the sun. Potential side effects include hyperpigmentation of the skin, blisters, or burns that can cause serious scars on your body. I recommend not using phototoxic oils on any skin that will be directly exposed to sunlight or UV rays, especially during the summertime. Wait at least twelve to seventy-two hours before directly exposing your skin post-application. Extreme care should be used with Bergamot (the worst offender), Lemon, Lime, Grapefruit, Petitgrain, Wild Orange, or any cold-pressed citrus oil. Cold-pressed means that the oils come directly from the rinds, so their potency is hard core. Always be sure to dilute them before applying topically.

Potentially phototoxic oils include Angelica, Anise, Bergamot, Bitter Orange, Celery/Celery Leaf/Celery Seed, Coriander, Cumin, Dill, Fig Leaf Absolute, Ginger, Grapefruit, Lemon, Lemon Verbena, Lime, Mandarin Orange, Orange, Tagetes, Tangerine, Wild Orange, and Yuzu.

Top 15 Essential Oils for Hormonal Balance

#1 BASIL (*Ocimum basilicum*)
Primary Chemical Constituent(s): Linalool
Properties: Calming/Soothing

#2 BERGAMOT (*Citrus bergamia*)
Primary Chemical Constituent(s): Limonene, linalyl acetate
Properties: Uplifting/Energizing
Safety Precautions:
Extremely phototoxic! Avoid direct sunlight and UV rays for a minimum of twelve to seventy-two hours after topical application.

#3 CEDARWOOD (*Juniperus virginiana*)

Primary Chemical Constituent(s): alpha-cedrene, cedrol, thujopsene

Properties: Grounding/Balancing

#4 CLARY SAGE (*Salvia sclarea*)

Primary Chemical Constituent(s): Linalyl acetate, linalool

Properties: Calming/Soothing

#5 GERANIUM (*Pelargonium graveolens*)

Primary Chemical Constituent(s): Citronellol, citronellyl formate, geraniol

Properties: Calming/Soothing

#6 LAVENDER (*Lavandula angustifolia*)

Primary Chemical Constituent(s): Linalool, linalyl acetate

Properties: Calming/Soothing

#7 LEMON (*Citrus limon*)

Primary Chemical Constituent(s): Limonene, beta-pinene, gamma-terpinene

Properties: Uplifting/Energizing

Safety Precautions:

Phototoxic! Always dilute prior to topical application; avoid direct sunlight and UV rays up to twelve hours after topical application.

#8 NEROLI (*Citrus × aurantium*)

Primary Chemical Constituent(s): Linalool, linalyl acetate, nerolidol

Properties: Calming/Soothing

#9 PEPPERMINT (*Mentha piperita*)

Primary Chemical Constituent(s): Menthol, menthone, 1,8-cineole

Properties: Uplifting/Energizing

#10 ROSEMARY (*Rosmarinus officinalis*)

Primary Chemical Constituent(s): 1,8-cineole, beta-pinene, camphor

Properties: Renewing and Grounding/Balancing

Safety Precautions:

Caution if epileptic, or if you have high blood pressure or a bleeding disorder.

#11 THYME *(Thymus vulgaris)*

    Primary Chemical Constituent(s): Thymol, para-cymene, gamma-terpinene

    Properties: Grounding/Balancing

#12 TURMERIC *(Curcuma longa)*

    Primary Chemical Constituent(s): Ar-turmerone, turmerone

    Properties: Grounding/Balancing

#13 YLANG YLANG *(Cananga odorata)*

    Primary Chemical Constituent(s): Germacrene, caryophyllene

    Properties: Calming/Soothing

#14 YARROW *(Achillea millefolium)*

    Primary Chemical Constituent(s): Punicic acid, beta-caryophyllene, chamazulene

    Properties: Calming/Soothing

#15 VITEX *(Vitex agnus-castus)*

    Primary Chemical Constituent(s): 1,8-cineole, sabinene, beta-caryophyllene

    Properties: Renewing and Grounding/Balancing

Top 5 Must-Have Essential Oils for Perimenopause

1. Clary Sage
2. Geranium
3. Lavender
4. Rosemary
5. Yarrow

Top 5 Must-Have Essential Oils for Menopause and Beyond

1. Clary Sage
2. Geranium
3. Peppermint
4. Turmeric
5. Ylang Ylang

PART II

Using Nutrition, Supplementation, Essential Oils, and Natural Remedies to Address Your Perimenopausal and Menopausal Symptoms

Chapter 4

Stress, the Silent Killer

At age forty-nine, Susan was having a hard time. As she explained to me: "It feels like I don't have any emotional resilience anymore. I snap at everyone and it's impacting my relationships at the office and at home. I wish everyone could understand that I am going nonstop all day long and I can't even get through the endless to-do list. There are days I don't even come close and I just want to cry looking at my list at night. And I am so tired by three p.m. every day, even on the weekend. No day is safe anymore, I feel stressed twenty-four/seven and I'm out of solutions."

Preliminary hormone tests showed Susan had long-standing chronic stress. Her cortisol levels were dysregulated, low in the morning (when they should have been high) and continuing to stay low in the afternoon and evening. All this was exacerbated by her age and the fact that her periods were now not as regular as they'd once been: She was perimenopausal.

My recommendations for Susan were as follows:

- Five daily supplements: a multivitamin, methylated B vitamin complex, 1,000 mg vitamin C, 400 mg magnesium glycinate, and 2,000 mg omega-3 fatty acids to lower stress levels and inflammation and increase energy.
- Substituting matcha for coffee. The L-theanine in green tea reduces stress without causing sedation.

- Holy basil tea in the evening before bed to reduce feelings of worry and stress.
- Green smoothie with protein, healthy fats, and fiber for breakfast instead of coffee and toast.
- 20-minute Morning Ritual: Daily Self-Care Journal (page 266) and Mindfulness Meditation.
- 5- to 10-minute meditations in the morning and afternoon with a meditation app (Headspace or Stop, Breathe & Think app).
- For afternoon slumps use the Instant Motivation Rollerball Blend (page 132).
- For sleep, Deep Sleep Diffuser Blend (page 101) in a diffuser two hours before bed. Lavender on her neck and feet before going to bed.

Within a month, Susan sent me an update. "Dr. Mariza, it's hard to believe, but so much has shifted for me. My occasional energy slumps are easily fixed with oils, so I have them with me each day at work. Magnesium has changed my life. I am sleeping better at night and it takes the edge off before going to bed. Even though I was really resistant to starting the morning rituals, I knew I needed a radical change. I needed to finally focus on myself, even for twenty minutes in the morning. I started with a five-minute meditation and I worked up to ten minutes in the morning and five minutes in the afternoon during my work break. Clearing my mind helped me let go of obligations. I feel less stressed and my family immediately noticed the change in my mood at night. I felt like I had more to give them. I will be continuing my morning rituals, supplements, and oils. I think I may try to bring coffee back next month, but for now matcha is working its magic and I feel pretty good."

What's Going On

Stress comes in several forms: emotional stress, stress related to trauma, and physical stress. Emotional stress can be caused by chronic worry, feeling overwhelmed, without the ability to relax, and emotionally taxing or devastating events, such as losing a job, bankruptcy, an accident or injury, or the loss of a loved one.

Trauma-related stress is caused by an experience that overwhelms us, shatters our sense of security, and makes us feel frightened and vulnerable. This could be a onetime event, such as a theft or a car crash, or one that occurs repeatedly such as bullying, domestic violence, or childhood abuse and neglect. Serious illness, intrusive medical procedures, and natural and man-made disasters can also result in trauma.

Physical stress comes from not getting enough sleep (your body can't restore its reserves) and poor nutrition, which deprives you of energy. Environmental toxins also cause physical stress in that they put a strain on your organs, tissues, and cells. Illness, especially chronic illness, is a main driver of physical stress, too.

No matter what type of stress you're dealing with, it triggers your stress response and your HPA axis. Cortisol floods your system, raising your blood pressure and heart rate while boosting blood sugar for an energy kick. Systems nonessential for your immediate survival such as digestion and reproduction are slowed way down. You are in full-on fight-or-flight mode. Once the stress has been managed, the body's systems return to normal and rebalance. Our stress response is in place to protect us in the short term from acute stress, not to stay in survival mode 24/7.

But many of us are *living* in survival mode. Stressors are no longer the occasional saber-tooth tiger of our prehistoric days, but everything from an urgent text from work to a bumper-to-bumper commute. Processed food is everywhere and sleep is hard to get. Our bodies are constantly on guard. This is exhausting to the body—it takes a lot of energy to always be in survival mode—eroding our resilience, our immediate capacity to respond to stress; and our metabolic reserve, our long-term capacity to withstand stress. This spells disaster for women in perimenopause and menopause. Especially when we tell ourselves the lie that we are fueled by the stress. Our mind tries to write a check our bodies can't cash!

Is Stress Impacting Your Health and Hormones?

Are you addicted to stress? For many years I was. I thought stress was my superpower, fueling my drive and ambition to be the best doctor, daughter, sister, wife, and friend. I was your typical Rushing Woman, cramming as much as possible into each day, trying to be everything to everybody, and adding more and more to my plate—until my plate became a massive unmanageable platter. Yet I still found myself stressing about not doing enough, especially for other people.

I have found that often we don't even know we are experiencing stress. So, to create some awareness regarding your perceived stress, I want to invite you to do this stress assessment with me. Read over the list below.

- You find yourself saying, "I gotta go. I am running late," or "I am super busy."
- You find that your calendar is consistently overscheduled.
- You find that you're upset when things change unexpectedly.
- You feel irritated when obligations stack up and you are not able to handle them.
- You often feel like things are not going your way.
- You often feel overwhelmed by the lack of support you have each day.
- You wake up feeling like there isn't enough time in the day to get everything done.
- You go to bed worrying that you did not finish your to-do list.
- You frequently feel like there's always something more you should be doing right now.
- You find yourself craving a salty or sugary snack in the middle of the day.

- You feel wired and tired.
- You feel like you have a low stress tolerance.
- You feel exhausted in the middle of the day, at three or four p.m.
- You can't turn off all the thoughts in your mind when trying to go to sleep.
- You rarely feel like you are completely on top of things.
- You get sick easily: Coughs and infections take a long time to resolve.
- You have no willpower when it comes to food.
- You need caffeine to function during the day.

If you answered yes to three or fewer, good news! You are experiencing normal stress levels that occur in everyday life.

If you answered yes to four or more, you are mostly likely experiencing an overactivation of your stress response system.

Did many of those statements feel familiar? If so, you're a lot like I was and many other women out there. Chronic stress, occurring over prolonged periods, throws our body and hormones out of whack, causing a litany of miserable symptoms whether or not you're yet in menopause!

The Perimenopause/Menopause Connection

The list of ways stress can make us sick looks a lot like the most common symptoms of perimenopause and menopause: weight gain, low libido, digestive issues, anxiety and depression, and more. That's because the majority of the problems that we women have, especially those related to hormones and perimenopause and menopause symptoms, originate with stress and an imbalance in the HPA axis.

Midlife is one of the most stressful times there is. Demands on your time and energy are at an all-time high from partners, kids, parents, and colleagues. And in perimenopause or menopause, we're also dealing with our body's physical changes and what they mean for us. Now, more than ever, we need to lower our stress burden, emotionally and physically, and get off the HPA axis dysfunction hamster wheel. It is one of the best moves you can make to regulate your hormones and significantly reduce or resolve your perimenopause or menopause symptoms.

Why It's Happening

There's a lot going on when it comes to stress. Pretty much anything that takes your body out of homeostasis, or stability, causes it. That's why supporting your body's natural hormonal balance and reducing inflammation, through diet, exercise, and self-care, eases stress. Whether you're stressed because you're working long hours, dealing with a difficult relationship, raising a child on your own, or racing around like a classic Rushing Woman, these are some of the hormonal imbalances at play and the most common yet overlooked root causes.

Too Much Cortisol/HPA Axis Dysfunction

Cortisol is vital for good health, affecting many different functions in the body. It's so important, most cells in the body have cortisol receptors. Cortisol helps control blood sugar levels and blood pressure, regulates metabolism, reduces inflammation, and assists with memory formulation. And it springs into action due to acute stress, preparing us for fight or flight. But chronically elevated cortisol levels are bad news, disrupting the whole HPA axis and stressing the body.

Over time, cells become cortisol resistant, and the natural rise and fall of cortisol, rising in the morning to wake you up and falling in the evening as you wind down, gets messed up, ruining your sleep-wake cycle and the other processes regulated by your circadian rhythm. You're primed for tired-but-wired fatigue, insomnia, skin issues, mood swings, muscle tension, low libido, fatty, sugary food cravings, weight gain, and digestive distress. Inflammation fires up and your immune system is compromised, setting you up for chronic conditions and autoimmune diseases. Balancing cortisol and resetting the wayward HPA is the key to getting stress under control and restoring hormonal balance.

Dysregulated Insulin and Blood Sugar

Insulin and cortisol counterbalance each other, so when cortisol is dysregulated, insulin is impacted, too. Elevated insulin promotes insulin resistance, inflammation, moodiness, sleep issues, sugar and carb cravings, and increased belly fat from all of that extra sugar. Insulin spikes also increase the destruction of the thyroid in people with autoimmune thyroid disease.

Insulin regulates your blood sugar levels, and if these become erratic or chronically too high or too low, it places significant stress on your body. If left unchecked, high blood sugar can lead to serious health issues: heart disease, stroke, and eye, nerve, and kidney damage. Low blood sugar leaves you irritable, anxious, foggy-brained, hangry, and intensely craving more carbohydrates (usually in the form of refined sugars) or caffeine to bring your blood sugar levels back up to normal as quickly as possible. Dysregulated blood sugar makes it tough to sleep, and a lack of restorative sleep is a major stress on the body. Eating to stabilize blood sugar is one of the best things you can do to lower stress.

Diet High in Processed and Inflammatory Foods/Gut Issues

Your gut is the most important gateway to your overall health. The gut makes and regulates hormones and neurotransmitters involved in nearly every bodily function, including estrogens, thyroid hormones, melatonin, and serotonin. It contains most of your immune system and it's your second brain, in direct connection with your brain and therefore highly influencing your moods and sense of emotional well-being. Eating a diet high in processed food, sugars, carbs, and inflammatory foods, such as gluten and dairy, stresses your gut. It alters your gut microbiome, upsetting the balance of "good" bacteria and "bad" bacteria, compromising your ability to properly digest and absorb the vitamins and nutrients from your food and metabolize hormones, such as estrogen. An imbalanced microbiome and an inflammatory diet can poke holes in the intestinal barrier, allowing toxins to seep from inside the intestine into the bloodstream, initiating an immune system response to attack those toxins. If the gut remains leaky, and toxins keep spilling out, inflammation—another devastating stressor on the body—goes wild.

Circadian Rhythm Dysfunction/Poor Sleep Hygiene

Our biological processes, the rise and fall of our hormones, when we sleep and eat, even the bacteria in our microbiome, operate on an internal twenty-four-hour cycle influenced in large part by light, called our circadian rhythm. When we live in sync with this cycle, resting at night and being active during the day, for example, our body is in balance. We throw off this cycle by staying up late at night, getting too much artificial light, especially blue light from screens, in the evening, not being exposed to enough sunlight during the day, or eating at all hours of the day and night.

One of the most obvious results of circadian rhythm dysfunction is trouble sleeping. You're revved up at night and can't wind down even though you're tired, and then struggle to get out of bed in the morning. Not enough or poor sleep increases inflammation, depresses the immune system, promotes insulin and blood sugar dysregulation, impairs brain function, and much, much more. It puts a lot of pressure on the body to try to compensate.

Toxins

Environmental toxins, pesticides, solvents, heavy metals, even the preservatives and artificial flavorings in processed food, stress the body, damaging nearly all of your organs and systems, throwing your digestive tract, liver, and kidneys into detox overwhelm, and causing inflammation. Toxins even damage DNA, increasing the rate of cell aging and degeneration, and can activate or suppress our gene expression in negative ways.

What You Can Do to Calm Stress

It's impossible to completely get rid of stress. The goal of stress management is to identify your root cause stressors and reduce their negative impact on you. Learn to notice the signs that you are becoming emotionally stressed—for me, it's sweating the small stuff. For you, it might be snapping at a friend or tension in your neck. When those telltale signs pop up, you need to deal with the stress proactively rather than ignoring it.

Incorporating essential oils on a daily basis will help you manage the inevitable effects of stress and keep your body from slipping into a chronic stress loop. Science strongly demonstrates the aromatherapeutic effect of linalool in essential oils like Lavender and Clary Sage, as well as the calming and grounding effects of the others in this list (page 82). I recommend choosing one or two favorites for a daily ritual, while also having a go-to blend in your purse for those moments when you need immediate calm. The following essential oil blends, supplements, herbs, and self-care rituals will help you de-stress. Use these in concert with the Makeover Program in Part III to create ease and grace. Also turn to the chapters on sleep and digestion for more help targeting those root causes. And seek professional support, especially if you're dealing with trauma.

How to Identify Perceived Stress Triggers

Awareness of your stressors is the number one tool to reduce chronic perceived stress and change the way your brain perceives external environmental stressors. It's key to train yourself to monitor for signs that your stress response system has been activated. For example, you may notice:

- physiological signs—feeling hot and sweaty; face flushing; shallower breathing; racing hearbeat.
- a rush of anxiety, or your mind racing.
- being stuck in a fearful way of thinking, unable to see a different perspective.
- feeling panicky and wanting to act impulsively.
- treating friends and family in a less-than-ideal way.

Once you notice that you are triggered, the next thing is to stop what you are doing, take a pause, and take charge of your physical state. It's time to change your physiology.

If you are in fight-or-flight mode, the best way to calm down is to slow down your breathing or to breathe into your belly. This puts the brakes on your stress response system. Your brain quickly senses it's safe and sends signals throughout the system to stop producing cortisol and return to its baseline.

And here's a proactive option: Send the brain safety signals even before you ever find yourself experiencing stress or panic. Safety signals take the form of self-care such as meditation, a walk outside, or deep breathing a calming essential oil. They are powerful and effective ways to tell the brain that everything is okay and there is nothing to panic about.

Top 5 Essential Oils for Stress

1. Bergamot
2. Cedarwood
3. Clary Sage
4. Frankincense
5. Lavender

Essential Oil Blends

Diffuser Blends

Zen Out Diffuser Blend

2 drops Cedarwood essential oil
2 drops Tangerine essential oil
2 drops Lavender essential oil

Chill Out Diffuser Blend

2 drops Lavender essential oil
2 drops Roman Chamomile essential oil
2 drops Sandalwood essential oil
2 drops Clary Sage essential oil

Grounding Diffuser Blend

2 drops Green Mandarin essential oil
2 drops Clary Sage essential oil
I drop Frankincense or Cedarwood essential oil

Personal Inhaler Blends

Reset and Restore Inhaler Blend

4 drops Bergamot essential oil
4 drops Ylang Ylang essential oil
4 drops Lavender essential oil
3 drops Grapefruit essential oil

Centered Calm Inhaler Blend

4 drops Clary Sage essential oil
4 drops Wild Orange essential oil
3 drops Frankincense essential oil
2 drops Cedarwood essential oil

Aromatic Sprays

Ease and Grace Spritz

10 drops Tangerine essential oil
8 drops Lavender essential oil
5 drops Clary Sage essential oil
Distilled water or witch hazel

Stress Release Room Spritz

20 drops Frankincense essential oil
20 drops Bergamot essential oil
20 drops Lavender essential oil
Distilled water or witch hazel

Rollerball Blends

De-Stress Rollerball Blend

12 drops Lavender essential oil
9 drops Copaiba essential oil
9 drops Wild Orange essential oil
Carrier oil of choice

Apply to pulse points and bottoms of feet for instant stress relief.

Ease Tension Rollerball Blend

10 drops Lavender essential oil
10 drops Clary Sage essential oil
10 drops Peppermint essential oil
Carrier oil of choice

Apply to pulse points or any areas affected by tension to release pent-up stress. Inhale deeply for a quick recharge.

Keep It Moving Rollerball Blend

8 drops Bergamot essential oil

8 drops Peppermint essential oil

6 drops Ylang Ylang essential oil

4 drops Wild Orange essential oil

Carrier oil of choice

Apply behind ears, on wrists, and to the back of neck while deeply inhaling to calmly focus and motivate you to carry on.

Stress-Reducing Supplements and Herbal Remedies

Stress-reducing supplements seem to be lurking around every corner these days. But how can you tell which ones actually work?

When you're reaching for supplements to address your stress, you want to be sure they are getting to the root of the problem. Whether that is addressing hormone imbalances, supporting your brain's calming neurotransmitters, allowing you to get higher-quality sleep, or easing any of the other possible root causes, understanding what's causing the stress in your body is the key to supplement success.

In addition to the supplements I recommend as part of the 21-Day Hormone Makeover Program (page 257), consider adding the following:

Supplements

ESSENTIALLY WHOLE® CALM & RESTORE

GABA (gamma-aminobutyric acid) is one of the primary calming neurotransmitters in your body. Calm & Restore provides a bioavailable form of GABA derived from a natural fermentation process to help outweigh heightened stress responses and help you feel more calm, focused, and in control.

L-THEANINE (100–200 MG/DAY)

Supporting your brain's calming neurotransmitters is one of the best ways to calm an overactive stress response. L-theanine supplements are clinically proven to reduce feelings of stress and promote higher-quality sleep by supporting the production of calming neurotransmitters and suppressing the ones that rev you up.

Herbs

ASHWAGANDHA (300–500 MG/DAY) AND RHODIOLA (START AT 50 MG/DAY AND STEADILY INCREASE UNTIL YOU ACHIEVE DESIRED RESULTS, BUT NOT TO EXCEED 680 MG/DAY)

These are two of my favorites to help take the edge off mental and physical feelings of stress. Whatever type of stress you're facing, these two adaptogens support healthy stress responses by regulating your nervous system. Beyond just reducing your feelings of stress, they go to the root to stabilize the hormones that could be contributing to your frazzled state.

Please note that if you're sensitive to nightshades, these can be a trigger for some people, so use caution when implementing them into your routine.

LEMON BALM (300–1,200 MG/DAY)

This herb activates the calming neurotransmitters in your brain to enable you to wind down, feel less stress, and get better sleep. Research even suggests that it works as well as some relaxant medications—but without the negative side effects.

Dr. Mariza's Hormone-Loving Rituals and Protocols

Morning Ritual

Since I discovered the power of essential oils, I have always started my day with a specific Morning Ritual that helps me charge into my day with intention, purpose, and love. Designing one that works for you depends on your personal needs in the morning balanced with the time you have to give yourself. I recommend waking at the same time each morning so that your body knows when to expect to rise, which supports your hormonal needs by balancing circadian rhythms. Know, too, that how you approach the world greatly influences your power for change and purpose. Your body will know what to expect each and every day, allowing you to move purposely and powerfully into the world. It is all about giving your body what it needs, which goes beyond nutrition.

Here are the four steps of my Morning Ritual that I recommend following each morning to live your best life.

#1 SELF-LOVE: SELF-AFFIRMATION WITH DIFFUSION AND DEEP BREATHING

Diffuse—Beginning your day with a diffuser blend will tap the healing power of essential oils, aromas your body will come to associate with a new beginning each day. I recommend firing up your diffuser first thing with my energizing Abundance Blend, and allowing it to fill the room as you repeat positive affirmations while breathing deeply.

Abundance Diffuser Blend
2 drops Frankincense or Sandalwood
2 drops Wild Orange
1 drop Peppermint

Positive Affirmations—Find affirmations that keep you poised, present, and powerful. I combine a few of these nuggets to create an affirmation I write in my journal each day.

- Today is a great day.
- I am enough.
- I am worthy.
- I deserve happiness.
- I deserve love.
- I am energized and inspired.
- I am worthy of feeling good.
- I define my own success.
- My day unfolds with ease and grace.
- People support me throughout the day.
- I am a positive influence on the world.

Another little tip: Record yourself saying your affirmations on a day you feel ultra-confident. Then play it back for yourself whenever a moment of stress threatens to derail your day. Your own voice giving you your own unique personal mantras holds amazing power!

Deep Breathing—To employ effective deep breathing, start by paying attention to your diaphragm, a powerful weapon in creating calm. As you slowly inhale through your nose for a count of eight, your stomach should pull outward from your belly button as if an invisible string were slowly tugging on it as your diaphragm fills with air. Then slowly begin to exhale for a count of six, with an invisible string pulling the belly button backward through your body, pushing all of the air back out through your mouth. Pause and hang in the space at the bottom, repeating your deep breathing for six, or more, breaths.

When I am breathing deeply, I love imagining myself taking in all of the positivity and energy from the outside. Then I exhale out all of the stress and tension I am holding. I continue to breathe deeply until I feel relaxed, nonresistant, and clear.

#2 START WITH GRATITUDE: JOURNALING WITH MEDITATION AND PRAYER

Beginning your morning with a gratitude practice will enable you to appreciate the power of pause and center your mind while recognizing those things for which you are most thankful. I like to journal what I'm grateful for in my Daily Self-Care Journal (see page 266) but feel free to journal in whatever way helps you to start your day with intention and purpose.

In addition, I recommend setting up a sacred space in your home for meditation and prayer. These practices release endorphins into the bloodstream, flooding you with happiness that will permeate throughout your day.

#3 NOURISH YOUR BODY: PROPER HYDRATION, NUTRITION, AND MOVEMENT

MORNING HYDRATION

Drinking water should be a top priority for you, especially in the morning when you are dehydrated from a lack of liquid intake overnight. First thing, you need to hydrate with 16 to 32 ounces of water to give you mental clarity that boosts energy and sets your body in the right mood for the day. I personally love water infusions for an extra flavor boost. Water infusions do well if you prep them the night before so you are not rushing to make one in the morning. Here is one of my favorite infusions. You can find more water infusions in Chapter 17.

Detox and Recharge Water Infusion

$1/2$ cup organic blueberries
$1/2$ cup organic cucumbers, sliced into rounds
1 organic lemon, sliced into rounds
$1 1/2$ quarts filtered water

In a small glass bowl, muddle the blueberries. Place slices of cucumber and lemon into a 2-quart glass pitcher and add the berry mixture on top.

Slowly pour in your water, refrigerating for 3 to 5 hours (or overnight) before serving either warm or over ice. This can sit for up to 3 days in your refrigerator!

In addition to water and infusions, start your morning with warm lemon water, bone broth, herbal tea, or a warm matcha latte.

PROPER NUTRITION

Truth: My green smoothie habit helped me kick my midmorning coffee/candy addiction. In over a decade of educating on women's health, I have learned one important fact: Food is foundational. Nourishing your body in the morning with whole foods is the best way to ensure energy and focus for the entire day. I recommend that your breakfast contain protein, fiber, and healthy fats so that you feel nourished and full until lunch. If you don't have time to make breakfast, whip up a smoothie. My husband Alex and I have a smoothie station in our kitchen with our blender, protein powder, fiber, and favorite essential oils with frozen greens and berries on hand in the freezer. It takes us five minutes to make two 16-ounce smoothies. My Hormone Love Smoothie (page 310) is one of my favorites.

POWER IN MOVEMENT

Honoring your body with movement will help you find calm amid stress and keep your hormones balanced. Any movement is better than no movement at all, but I recommend finding the one that re-laxes *and* energizes. For me, nature speaks to my soul, so a brisk ten- to fifteen-minute walk in the morning or some time during the day soothes and reinvigorates my mind.

#4 SET AN INTENTION: DAY PLANNING AND FLEXIBILITY

If you don't have a personal schedule or day planner, I highly recommend getting one or using an app on your phone. Many of us become stressed by unpredictability, and planning your day alleviates the worry of forgetting important to-dos. I spend time planning my day so that I am living my day by design, not default, allowing me to maximize my time and focus on the things that really matter. And allow yourself the grace of flexibility. Remind yourself that you can say no to anything that's not in alignment with your emotional well-being.

And if you have to do something that causes you stress, prepare yourself with aromatherapy, positive affirmations, and deep breathing to keep your calm.

Midday Stress-Busting Rituals

When moments of craziness threaten to derail you, there are some powerful rituals that I employ to keep my mind present and my emotions on an even keel. See if these work for you, too.

Aroma Power—Choose your favorite single oil or rollerball blend and take a deep inhale to de-stress and refuel. Roll it on your pulse points and sit with the aroma for a minute.

Mindfulness Meditation—Even a one-minute deep-breathing meditation or prayer break to reset your mind and soul can recharge your body and refocus your intent.

Hydrate—The body often mistakes thirst for hunger, so before you go slam a bar or knock back caffeine, try drinking 4 to 8 ounces of water and give yourself ten minutes for it to kick into action.

Chapter 5

Sleep Issues

Christina, age fifty-two, reached out to me after trying endless remedies to help her sleep through the night. Since turning fifty, she had struggled to stay asleep, and some nights she tossed and turned until she finally got out of bed and worked for an hour before trying to go back to sleep. Christina disclosed that her sleep issues were affecting everything in her life. She shared in an email: "I can't think straight some days because I am so tired. I know my work is suffering. The words just blur on the computer screen. I am putting on weight, despite changing nothing in my diet. I know it's my lack of sleep. And I am beginning to feel depressed because I am so tired. Anything you can do to help; I am feeling hopeless."

Christina was entering menopause and suffering from chronic fatigue, low cortisol in the morning, and low metabolic resilience due to poor sleep quality.

My recommendations were as follows:

- Four daily supplements: a multivitamin, 100 mg L-theanine, 400 mg magnesium glycinate, and 2,000 mg omega-3 fatty acids to lower stress levels and support brain function.
- Two sleep supplements: 180–250 mg valerian and 1 capsule Essentially Whole® Zen Sleep before bed.
- Substituting holy basil tea for coffee in the afternoon and evening.

- For afternoon work slumps, Energy Restored Rollerball Blend (page 132) to stay focused and sharp.
- For sleep, she should use the Deep Sleep Diffuser Blend (page 101) in a diffuser, two hours before bed. I also recommended that she apply Lavender and Vetiver on her neck and feet before going to bed.
- A 20-minute Nighttime Ritual, including a sleep meditation, before bed to relax the mind before sleep.
- 15-minute afternoon nature walks five times a week to boost energy and good-feeling emotions.

Three weeks later I reached out to Christina to follow up on her progress. She was excited to report: "I felt like I made a lot of changes to improve my sleep and energy levels and they are paying off. I didn't realize that I needed to make changes throughout my day to get my sleep back on track. I am happy to report that most nights I am getting seven hours and I am not getting up to work in the middle of the night. If I do wake up, I apply my oils and do a sleep meditation and fall back asleep. I am focused at work and slowly losing the extra pounds I gained. I am committed to my night routine, supplements, and new habits. I can see that they have more benefits than just sleep for me."

What's Going On

Are you exhausted at night but unable to shut down the mental chatter and relax enough to sleep? Do you get up several times during the night and struggle to get back to sleep? Do you wake up feeling like you've never slept?

Our buzzing brains, endless to-do lists, jam-packed schedules, and myriad responsibilities make good sleep a challenge. (Not to mention computer screens, snoring partners, and restless pets!) Add in hot flashes, night sweats, and an overactive bladder—all common in peri-menopause and menopause—and your sleep is likely disrupted on a regular basis.

According to recent findings by the Centers for Disease Control and Prevention (CDC), a whopping half of perimenopausal women wake up feeling exhausted four or more days each week. For some women, sleep improves after menopause and the hormonal roller coaster levels out, but for others new sleep challenges arise, such as an increasing likelihood of sleep apnea, compromising their ability to get good sleep. That same CDC study found that more than half of women in menopause—55.1 percent—are sleeping poorly enough to wake feeling tired, not rested, four or more times a week. No wonder our hormones are imbalanced, our energy is zapped, and our tempers frayed!

Sleep is as essential as eating and breathing, giving our body and mind the time they need to rest and repair. Without it, our health and hormones suffer in significant ways. Poor sleep:

- increases chronic inflammation, a driver of nearly all chronic diseases.
- depresses the immune system, making us more susceptible to illness and chronic infections.
- promotes insulin resistance and impairs blood sugar balance. With lack of sleep, cells respond poorly to insulin, starving them of the glucose fuel they need to function and raising blood sugar levels. A 2015 study found that one night of sleep deprivation was as detrimental to insulin sensitivity as six months of eating a high-fat diet.
- contributes to weight gain by deregulating our "hunger hormones" leptin and ghrelin so we never feel full and are hungrier, leading to binge eating, late-night snacks, and cravings.
- compromises the repair of our muscles and other tissues. Human growth hormone (HGH) is released during sleep so our bodies can continue to grow and develop and we can heal damaged tissue. When we don't get enough sleep, our pituitary gland pumps out less of this vital hormone, increasing our risk of heart disease, obesity, diabetes, and mental health issues.
- impairs brain function, weakening our memory, judgment, concentration, and ability to problem-solve. Sleep is also when nasty toxic proteins are cleared out of the brain. A buildup of

these beta-amyloid proteins is associated with Alzheimer's disease.

Upgrading your sleep is one of the most effective ways to ease your path through perimenopause and menopause and lift your health in general. If you have a hard time remembering the last night you had at least seven hours of uninterrupted sleep that left you feeling refreshed and energized to start your day, you've come to the right place for some sleep TLC.

What's Restful Sleep, Anyway?

We all know the amount of sleep we get matters. According to the National Sleep Foundation (NSF), adults ages twenty-six to sixty-four need seven to nine hours of sleep, while adults sixty-five years and older require seven to eight hours. Not getting sufficient shut-eye means you're pushing your body to run on less than it needs. But the *quality* of sleep matters, too. A panel of experts in conjunction with the NSF describe good sleep quality as:

- Sleeping for at least 85 percent of the total time you are in bed
- Falling asleep in 30 minutes or less
- Waking up no more than once per night
- Being awake for 20 minutes or less after initially falling asleep

Why It's Happening

Sleep regulates the release of many of our hormones, so not getting enough means trouble for hormone balance. In turn, hormonal changes, including fluctuating estrogen and progesterone, can wreak havoc on your sleep patterns. Whether you are waking up because of night sweats, you are having trouble falling asleep because your mind won't stop spinning, or you just don't feel rested, here are some of the hormone imbalances and root causes contributing to your sleep issues.

Low Estrogen

Estrogen promotes good-quality sleep, reducing awakenings during the night and the amount of time needed to fall asleep. The problem lies in fluctuating estrogen levels during perimenopause and low levels in menopause, which contribute to sleep issues and make us susceptible to hot flashes, night sweats, anxiety, and headaches that can interfere with sleep. Low estrogen also affects our circadian rhythm, the twenty-four-hour internal clock that regulates our sleep/wake cycle and body temperature, contributing to disrupted sleep. And less estrogen means we're less efficient at processing magnesium, an important mineral for sleep regulation.

Low Progesterone

Progesterone is a sleep-promoting "feel-good" hormone that keeps us calm while reducing anxiety and symptoms of depression. When progesterone levels are optimal, we are relaxed, fall asleep easily, and sleep well through the night. As progesterone declines during perimenopause and menopause, we may feel more anxious, hindering our ability to sleep, and we wake up more frequently during the night. Progesterone also helps us to breathe easily while we sleep, so low levels may contribute to an increased likelihood of sleep apnea and other breathing disruptions during the night.

Low Melatonin

Melatonin is often called the "sleep hormone" because it tells your body it's time to wind down, helping you to fall asleep easier. Melatonin production and release is directly tied to your circadian rhythm and the amount of light the pineal glands in your eyes are exposed to. Levels rise in the evening, as light decreases, making you drowsy. They stay elevated through the night, falling with sunrise and the increasing light of a new day. Melatonin in the body is barely detectable during daylight. If you're not making enough melatonin or your pineal gland isn't releasing it on cue in the evening because your environment is too brightly lit, you'll have a difficult time going to sleep and staying there.

Contrary to a widespread myth, melatonin levels don't decrease with age; in healthy adults they remain static over time. Low melatonin or a disrupted release schedule isn't due to age but other root causes, such as too much bright light at night, lack of exposure to natural light during the day, stress, and nutrient deficiencies.

Thyroid Hormone Imbalance

Your thyroid plays an incredibly important role regulating your metabolism, energy level, and other hormones. If your thyroid is malfunctioning, it can throw off everything, including your sleep.

In those with hypothyroidism, reproductive hormones such as estrogen and progesterone drop. A decrease in estrogen results in troubled sleep, while falling progesterone levels are likely the reason for a greater risk of developing sleep apnea. More frequent awakenings during the night result in lighter, poorer sleep. Elevated cortisol, a common symptom of an underactive thyroid, keeps your body and mind switched on and unable to doze off.

In the case of hyperthyroidism, an overactive thyroid revs up the body, making it hard to unwind. And an inability to adequately regulate body temperature can lead to night sweats.

Dysregulated Insulin and Blood Sugar

Insulin regulates blood sugar throughout the day and night. In the early morning, usually between four and eight a.m., we experience a surge in glucose to kick-start our day. This triggers the body to produce insulin to move the glucose into cells, keeping the blood sugar under control. If insulin is unable to do its job, either because the body isn't producing enough insulin or too much insulin has made the cells unable to use it correctly (insulin resistance), high blood sugar results. This sets us up for imbalanced blood sugar, meaning you fall into the sugar rush and crash cycle throughout the day. Late morning and early afternoon snack cravings are telltale signs of this rush-and-crash. By the time we're trying to fall asleep at night, we're in serious trouble.

High blood sugar is associated with poor sleep for several reasons. It gives you a burst of energy that can keep you awake, irritable, and unsettled. It can also wake you in the middle of the night with thirst or to use the bathroom. When your blood sugar is high, your kidneys work overtime to remove it through urination. Then once your blood sugar inevitably drops, it may fall too low, causing you to wake too early with hunger, chills, sweating, or restlessness.

Eating and hydrating for stable blood sugar all day—not just before bed—will help you sleep better at night.

Stress

Any type of stress makes it difficult to fall asleep and stay asleep, so it doesn't help that this time of life is packed with stressors, from work and home to relationships and health. We're also more prone to anxiety and depression, both of which can add to our stress and steal our sleep. Pushing ourselves to be everything to everybody each and every day, we're exhausted and yet unable to drift off at the end of the day.

Under chronic stress, your nervous and endocrine systems are on 24/7 alert, ready to deal with any danger coming your way. Your blood pressure is up and your digestive system is suppressed, causing upset stomach, pain, and bloating. Muscles become tense, contributing to headaches and neck strain. Elevated cortisol may cause you to crave more fatty foods, promoting heartburn and acid reflux. Everything about your body in nonstop crisis mode makes it tough to get good sleep. Does that pattern sound familiar? Lack of sleep then becomes one more stressor you sincerely do not need.

For good-quality, restful sleep, it's not enough for us to simply unwind in the evening (though it is essential!). We must also lower the burden of chronic stress keeping your body in a constant state of high alert.

Circadian Rhythm Dysfunction/Poor Sleep Hygiene

Our circadian rhythm is finely tuned to sync our eating, sleeping, blood sugar levels, and almost every other biological process with the twenty-four-hour cycle of light and dark, activity and rest. When we live in sync with this cycle, our hormones fluctuate to support productivity and alertness during the day and recovery and sleep at night. But when we live out of sync with this cycle, hormones such as melatonin, cortisol, and insulin are deeply affected. Sleep troubles enter into the mix and compromise our body's entire metabolic health, increasing our risk for diabetes, heart disease, and stroke.

Much of modern life makes it difficult to live in sync. Artificial lights, tablets and screens, irregular sleep schedules, and constant snacking can throw us off track. Not to mention nighttime working, texting, emailing, and checking social media. These all tell the brain and body it's time to be awake, not asleep. They do the exact opposite of what we need after a long day. Good sleep hygiene and established rituals and routines in our day, especially for when we sleep and eat, are key to supporting your natural circadian rhythm, getting restorative sleep, and balancing your hormones.

Sleep Apnea/Restless Legs Syndrome

Hot flashes and night sweats are most often blamed for ruining a good night's sleep, but sleep apnea and restless legs syndrome/Willis-Ekbom disease (RLS/WED) are culprits worth considering. In one study of menopausal women, more than half showed signs of one or both of these conditions.

Sleep apnea, a breathing disorder, is characterized by loud snoring, gasping, headaches, insomnia, and daytime fatigue. The risk of developing it increases with menopause, and according to research, women who experience severe hot flashes and night sweats are at nearly twice the risk than women with mild hot flashes or none at all. If you suspect this, talk to your partner or someone sleeping in your house. Chances are they can validate the snoring and sounds associated with sleep apnea.

Causing uncomfortable sensations in your legs with a powerful urge to move them, RLS/WED is most intense when you're relaxed or trying to sleep, leading to poor rest and daytime fatigue. Women are twice as likely to have it, and it generally worsens as you age. If you can't sit still without moving your legs or stretching your feet and ankles, you might be experiencing some nighttime problems as well without realizing that it is actually an issue.

Speak with your healthcare provider if you suspect you may have sleep apnea or RLS/WED. RLS can also be a sign of other autoimmune conditions such as lupus or celiac disease, so don't just dismiss it as normal for you.

What You Can Do to Support Good Sleep

The following essential oil blends, supplements, herbs, and self-care rituals are specifically designed to address the root causes by getting your stress levels in check and supporting a healthy circadian rhythm. Use these in concert with the Makeover Program in Part III to achieve the restorative sleep that you need and so richly deserve. Also turn to the chapters on stress and hot flashes, for more help targeting those root causes.

Top 5 Essential Oils for Sleep Support

1. Lavender
2. Vetiver
3. Cedarwood

4. Roman Chamomile
5. Ylang Ylang

Essential Oil Blends

Diffuser Blends

Relax and Restore Diffuser Blend

3 drops Roman Chamomile essential oil
2 drops Cedarwood essential oil
1 drop Lavender essential oil

Deep Sleep Diffuser Blend

2 drops Cedarwood essential oil
2 drops Lavender essential oil
2 drops Vetiver essential oil

Calm Mind Diffuser Blend

2 drops Clary Sage essential oil
2 drops Lavender essential oil
2 drops Ylang Ylang essential oil

Personal Inhaler Blends

Total Relaxation Inhaler Blend

3 drops Lavender essential oil
3 drops Ylang Ylang essential oil
3 drops Vetiver essential oil
2 drops Copaiba essential oil

Peaceful Mind Inhaler Blend

5 drops Lavender essential oil
4 drops Vetiver essential oil
4 drops Roman Chamomile essential oil
2 drops Ylang Ylang essential oil

Aromatic Sprays

Hot Flash Extinguisher Spritz

8 drops Peppermint essential oil
5 drops Lavender essential oil
2 drops Roman Chamomile essential oil
Distilled water or witch hazel

Spritz your body when hot flashes threaten to disrupt your sleep and lie back to allow the cooling sensation to relax your mind and body. Take care not to get it in your eyes!

Serene Sleep Spray

8 drops Lavender essential oil
8 drops Cedarwood essential oil
4 drops Vetiver essential oil
Distilled water or witch hazel

Spray your pillow and bedclothes as well as the air in your bedroom.

Rollerball Blends

Sweet Dreams Rollerball Blend

10 drops Lavender essential oil
8 drops Vetiver essential oil
4 drops Roman Chamomile essential oil
4 drops Ylang Ylang essential oil
Carrier oil of choice

Roll on the bottoms of your feet and on pulse points.

Mental Chatter Break Rollerball Blend

10 drops Lavender essential oil
8 drops Vetiver essential oil
5 drops Cedarwood essential oil
5 drops Clary Sage or Bergamot essential oil
Carrier oil of choice

Apply to the back of your neck and behind the ears to silence distracting mental chatter.

Tension Reliever Rollerball Blend

10 drops Lavender essential oil
6 drops Roman Chamomile essential oil
4 drops Clary Sage essential oil
2 drops Spearmint essential oil
Carrier oil of choice

Apply to the back of your neck and behind your ears, and to any other tense areas.

Grateful Meditation and Prayer Rollerball Blend

8 drops Frankincense essential oil
5 drops Bergamot essential oil
2 drops Ylang Ylang essential oil
Carrier oil of choice

Apply to pulse points.

Sleep-Supporting Supplements and Herbal Remedies

If you walk into a store looking for an over-the-counter drug to help you sleep—or even ask your doctor for something prescription strength—it's likely that the rest you'll get will come at a cost. Nasty side effects, addiction or chemical reliance, and next-day grogginess are par for the course when it comes to sleep aids. Luckily, they aren't your only option.

In addition to the supplements I recommend for everyone as part of the 21-Day Hormone Makeover Program (page 257), here are some of my go-tos to promote restful sleep naturally.

Supplements

GLYCINE (3–5 G BEFORE BED)

Research has found that glycine supplementation alleviates sleep issues such as trouble falling asleep or staying asleep while improving the quality of sleep and decreasing daytime tiredness. It can also help you feel sharper and more focused, thanks to better rest and improved neurotransmitter balance. I recommend combining glycine with magnesium in the form of magnesium glycinate before bed to support deep restful sleep.

L-THEANINE (100–200 MG/DAY)

If mental chatter, anxiety, stress, or racing thoughts are preventing you from getting the rest you need, L-theanine is a great natural way to bring calm and silence to your mental arena. It naturally supports your brain's ability to produce calming neurotransmitters that are responsible for sleep so you can wind down more easily and get higher-quality sleep.

ESSENTIALLY WHOLE® ZEN SLEEP

Zen Sleep provides a synergy of ingredients perfectly formulated to calm mental chatter and promote restful sleep, including chamomile and melatonin to help calm your mind and body and vitamin B6 to help your brain manage stress and promote restful sleep.

Herbs

ST. JOHN'S WORT (300 MG THREE TIMES A DAY [900 MG DAILY])

St. John's Wort is recognized as a natural way to boost your body's serotonin levels so you can get the rest you need and alleviate the fatigue and fogginess that come without it.

Please note that it can interact negatively with some prescriptions (especially ones designed for sleep or anxiety), so talk to your trusted practitioner before starting St. John's Wort if you take any other medications.

VALERIAN (450 MG/DAY)

Valerian is an herb with a rich history of promoting sleep and soothing anxiety. It works in much the same way as Valium or Xanax (but without the side effects): It allows your body to maintain elevated levels of calming neurotransmitters. Your amygdala is the part of your brain responsible for processing strong emotions and stress, and the compounds in valerian can help quiet this area in particular. It also contains powerful antioxidants that have sleep-enhancing properties.

MELATONIN (START WITH I MG AND INCREASE TO 3-5 MG AS NEEDED BEFORE BED)

When you think of herbal supplements for sleep, this is probably at the top of your list. A hormone that prepares you for sleep, melatonin is thrown off by any disruption to your circadian rhythm. Taking a supplement before bed is a natural way to restore the proper rhythm to your body and calm your mind as bedtime approaches.

CHAMOMILE, PASSIONFLOWER, AND/OR LAVENDER TEA

Drinking a cup of chamomile, passionflower, or lavender tea before bed is more than just a self-care ritual. The ingredients in this beverage contain compounds that naturally boost your brain's ability to wind down and rest. Be sure to select a brand without artificial additives, and if you want to add a sweetness, stevia is your best bet.

Dr. Mariza's Hormone-Loving Rituals and Protocols

Getting your stress under control is one of the best ways to promote good sleep. Follow the stress-releasing Hormone-Loving Rituals and Protocols in Chapter 4 and add this Nighttime Ritual for restful, supportive sleep.

Nighttime Ritual

Powering down in the evening shows that you appreciate what your body has done for you throughout the day and that you love it enough to treat it with gentleness and compassion. Your body will come to anticipate and rely on these rituals to help you enjoy your evening stress-free and eventually drift into a deep, restful sleep.

#1 POWER DOWN WITH A DIGITAL DETOX

Blue light emitted from your digital devices greatly disturbs your circadian rhythms and prevents your body from slipping into a restful sleep. Plus, it can continue to keep your mind firing on all cylinders when you really need some deep breathing, aromatherapy, and rest. Allow your brain to rest by putting your phone on silent (not just vibrate, *silent*) and resist the temptation to check it after eight p.m. (Or at least one hour prior to bedtime.) Read a good book, chill out with some slow tunes, or relax with a sleep meditation. Or better yet? Try a bath soak!

#2 DE-STRESS WITH BATH SOAKS

I love a good Epsom salt bath soak with relaxing essential oils. Use the recipes in this chapter or find your own favorite combination using about six drops of essential oil with two cups Epsom salts. Pair a relaxing playlist with your soak and prepare for a deep, restful sleep.

#3 DECOMPRESS WITH A SLEEP SANCTUARY

If your bedroom isn't an inviting and restful place, it is time to make it so! Blackout curtains work wonders for melatonin production, allowing sleep signals to fire. The right temperature is also key: 68–70°F (19–21°C) provides a heart-regulating sweet spot. Add a diffuser to your bedroom to diffuse your favorite sleep blend. Try Lavender or any of the essential oil recipes in this chapter.

The Good-Night HUG Ritual

This simple guided meditation focuses on three areas: Healing, Unwinding, and Gratitude.

H, Healing, means focusing on areas where you need healing grace and reflecting positively on areas where you have learned from this struggle.

U, Unwinding, means spending some time employing deep breathing while focusing on your intention for the day established in your Daily Self-Care Journal.

G, Gratitude, allows you to focus instead on the blessings from your day, while spending time to find the positive in overtly negative situations.

Chapter 6

Hot Flashes
and Night Sweats

Find yourself hot, sweaty, and miserable at the most inopportune moments? Or waking up drenched in sweat several times each night? You've probably heard your grandmother, mother, and aunts talking about the dreaded hot flashes and night sweats for years, and now, here you are. Indeed, hot flashes or night sweats are at the top of the menopausal complaint list!

Laura, age fifty-two, was no different. Hot flashes were disrupting her work. "As a family therapist, I see clients all day long and I can't begin to tell you how embarrassing it is to start pouring sweat in the middle of a session and then I experience extreme chills. I can't seem to get comfortable and it makes me feel so anxious, which I need to hide in front of my clients. No one wants a middle-aged, sweaty, anxious therapist. I run a fan constantly to decrease the severity of the flashes, but it only helps a little bit. I also noticed that they come on when I am feeling stressed about something."

Laura was suffering from hot flashes, stress, and occasional blood sugar imbalance.

My recommendations were as follows:

- Five daily supplements: a multivitamin, 400 IU vitamin E, 400 mg magnesium oxide, 500 mg myo-inositol, and 4 capsules

Essentially Whole® Hormone Balance to reduce hot flashes and stabilize blood sugar levels.

- The 21-Day Hormone Makeover Meal Plan to reset blood sugar levels, support liver detoxification, and support healthy hormone changes.
- For hot flashes, the Hot Flash Spritz (page 117) every hour.
- Peppermint and Lavender essential oils diffused during the day to reduce stress.
- Morning green smoothie with 1 scoop of maca (7–9 g).
- 5–10 minutes meditation in the morning and afternoon to reduce stress levels with a meditation app (Headspace App or Stop, Breathe & Think app).

Five weeks later, ten days after completing the 21-Day Program, Laura reached out to share her big wins. "I'm not running the fan constantly in my office! I am down to less than one hot flash a day, averaging three to four hot flashes a week. This is a massive improvement for me. My sweet tooth is under control after the 21-Day Program, and I think the green smoothie with maca is really helping. My hot flashes, if I have one, happen in the afternoon. And if I do have one, I quickly grab my hot flash spray to instantly cool me down. I keep the spray in my purse everywhere I go. I even use it on my friends. My other big realization was my stress levels. I didn't realize how stressed out I was, given my client load and everything else. No wonder I was feeling so anxious. The short meditations have cleared my mind and I feel more relaxed and centered. I know that has helped my hot flashes, too."

What's Going On

Hot flashes and night sweats are one of the most common issues I hear about from women in their late thirties on up. My mother's hot flashes were *epic,* with sudden waves of heat racing up her head and neck, leaving her skin red and blotchy, her face flushed, her heart racing, and her embarrassment soaring as work colleagues at the hospital couldn't help but notice her discomfort.

Lots of research supports their prevalence in women, especially those living in the United States. According to the Study of Women's Health Across the Nation (SWAN), a longitudinal study of women's health during middle age, 60 to 80 percent of women experience hot flashes at some point during the menopausal transition. These tend to begin during perimenopause and peak in occurrence and frequency in late perimenopause and early menopause. Yep, hot flashes may continue for several years after your last period. Some 40 percent of women sixty to sixty-five years old still have hot flashes. In addition, women who have had their ovaries removed and experience abrupt surgical menopause often have a sudden onset of severe hot flashes that continue for a longer stretch of time than women who undergo natural menopause.

You'd think with all of these women suffering and the amount of attention paid to hot flashes, we'd have a pretty solid handle on what causes them and how to find relief. Unfortunately, we don't have a definitive answer when it comes to exactly what causes hot flashes or a magic bullet for how to get rid of them. But it is not all doom and gloom. Quite the contrary! What we *do* know about hot flashes confirms that lifestyle plays a major role, and that means there's a lot we can do to adapt and get them under control or eliminate them entirely.

Here's what we know:

- **They're not just about estrogen.** We've been led to believe, and doctors have told us again and again, that hot flashes and night sweats are caused by falling estrogen levels. That's why when you mention hot flashes to most doctors, you'll be quickly handed a prescription for supplemental estrogen. But there's clearly way more going on. Sure, women with low estrogen experience hot flashes, but so do women with high or erratic levels. And so do women with low progesterone but normal estrogen levels. If it's all about estrogen, why do certain foods trigger hot flashes? Heck, men can get hot flashes if their testosterone level drops! All this to say, estrogen plays a part, but it is not onstage alone.

- **Mindset matters.** Women who hold negative beliefs about hot flashes, or say that they make them look foolish or weak, report more intense symptoms. And the real cracker: Women in other cultures with a more positive view of menopause than ours don't have nearly as much trouble with them—or trouble with them at all—as we do here in the United States.
- **Other hormones, such as insulin and cortisol, are big-time influencers.** As you'll see, an imbalance in these two hormones because of poor diet and stress may have even more of an influence on hot flashes than estrogen. That's why adaptive lifestyle changes are so fundamental to helping you feel better.

What's a Hot Flash, Anyway?

It sounds counterintuitive, but a hot flash (or hot flush) is your body's attempt at cooling itself off. It occurs when the hypothalamus, the part of the brain that regulates body temperature, senses the body is too hot and signals the body to let off the excess heat. One way it does this is by dilating the blood vessels in the skin of the chest, head, and neck. With the blood vessels opened more widely than usual, more blood flows through the area, making your skin feel hot and sticky and creating the telltale flush of red. The resulting perspiration and radiated heat works with the cooler air to lower your body temperature, just as sweat is supposed to do. That's why a hot flash is often followed by feeling chilled and clammy. One moment, you're on fire, and the next, you're freezing!

A hot flash can come on suddenly and last anywhere from thirty seconds to five minutes. In addition to the sudden rush of heat that moved from your chest to your neck to your face (and then the flush in the face and the sweat), you might also experience a tingling in your fingers, a racing or erratic heartbeat, or dizziness. Some women experience several in a day, while others have a few each week. My mom went from two to three per week to experiencing hot flashes two to three per day—and that's when she knew she needed to do something about them! Smoking, PMS, and obesity increase the likelihood of hot flashes, and overweight and obese women experience more severe ones, so reducing these triggers can greatly aid your body in restoring balance.

And a Night Sweat?

Hot flashes often occur while you're sleeping, and while the flash itself usually won't wake you up, the intense sweating—the night sweat—that follows to cool you down will. Some women lightly perspire, while others experience a drenching so severe they soak through their pajamas and sheets.

Hot Flash Triggers

Certain foods and circumstances—listed below—have been shown to trigger hot flashes, but each woman's triggers are different. By identifying your unique triggers, you can adapt to avoid them, thereby reducing the frequency of your hot flashes.

Hot drinks. That mug of scalding tea might be raising your body temperature just enough to trigger a hot flash. If you find this to be true for you, choose iced or room-temperature drinks instead.

Alcohol. Alcohol acts like sugar in the body, triggering a rise in blood glucose that can cause a hot flash. Also, your body widens the blood vessels that supply your skin when it's breaking down alcohol (you may have noticed this flush in yourself or others), which may invite a flash.

Spicy foods. Like alcohol, spicy foods, especially ones that contain the heat-producing compound capsaicin—for example, cayenne, chili powders, and hot peppers—expand your blood vessels. These are also in the nightshade family and can increase inflammation in the body.

Caffeine. It narrows blood vessels but raises your heart rate.

Emotions/Anxiety. Heightened anxiety and intense emotions rush the blood to the surface of our skin, prompting a sudden hot flash.

Jody (my mom): "The time I left my hot flash rollerball blend at home:"

> It was on my way to visit Mariza in Oakland. It was an hour flight up north from Southern California, but with extra travel and time at the airport, it was over two hours until I arrived. I packed quickly that day and I completely forgot to take my phytoestrogen supplement and hot flash rollerball blend with me. These two remedies had kept my hot flashes at bay for months and I wasn't going back. Luckily, I knew Mariza carried her hormone oils with her. The moment I landed, I grabbed my stuff and ran out to her car with my carry-on. Sure enough, there she was at the passenger pickup area, with her purse in the front seat. I opened the car door and before I said anything, I went into her purse and found her oil bag. I pulled out her Superwoman blend, similar to the one I used. I unbuttoned my jeans and applied it over my ovaries and put it in my pocket. I then looked up at her and said, "Hey, honey! I am keeping this for the weekend." That blend worked like a charm. No hot flashes all weekend long.

Why It's Happening

We're often quick to blame estrogen for hot flashes and night sweats. And it is a factor, but as I noted above, we can't blame it all on that one hormone. Cortisol and insulin levels are on the hook just as much, maybe even more so. In my experience, insulin resistance is the reason hot flashes persist—and why addressing the root causes of insulin resistance is a part of the Makeover Program.

Keep in mind, however, that there are other reasons you may experience hot flashes. Certain illnesses, such as anorexia nervosa, and medications, such as heart, blood pressure, sinus, and allergy medicines, painkillers, and estrogen-blocking drugs are potential culprits. Discussing this symptom with your trusted healthcare provider may enable you to find a solution.

Dysregulated Insulin and Blood Sugar/Insulin Resistance

Conventional medicine tells us there is no known root cause of hot flashes, but recent research indicates that it may be linked to insulin resistance. Basically, this means your body is not as efficient at delivering glucose (sugar) to your cells to use as energy, leading to spikes in the amount of glucose in your blood. Researchers have found that the frequency of hot flashes rise as blood sugar levels and the degree of insulin resistance rise. High blood sugar is very inflammatory, and this is responsible not only for hot flashes—and chronic inflammation may predispose women to more hot flashes—but can also contribute to fatigue, brain fog, pesky weight gain, and bleeding changes during your period. Fluctuating blood sugar levels are also connected to *more* hot flashes.

Riding the roller coaster of sugar highs and lows is definitely contributing to your hot flashes, so use the suggestions in this chapter and in the Hormone Makeover Program to stabilize your blood sugar and improve insulin sensitivity.

Wild Fluctuations of Estrogen and Progesterone

During perimenopause, changing hormonal levels can contribute to the incidence of hot flashes. Fluctuating levels of estrogen can cause your blood vessels to constrict or dilate, contributing to the onset of a hot flash. In addition, estrogen also plays a role in regulating body heat, with declining levels causing a reset of your internal thermo-stat. This triggers your body's cooling measures, like hot flashes, to be initiated sooner. Estrogen, especially estradiol, is also a potent anti-inflammatory, and lower levels may make some women more vulner-able to inflammation and hot flashes. Declining progesterone during perimenopause also affects your body's temperature control, and too little progesterone is linked to hot flashes.

Stress

No surprise that our old friend stress is at work here, too! In both perimenopausal and menopausal women, stress has been shown to make hot flashes worse. Women with the highest levels of stress were more than five times more likely than normally stressed women to report hot flashes. Five times!

Our flight-or-fight response, initiated in times of stress, kicks off the release of cortisol. When we're in survival mode chronically, as so many of us are, cortisol levels can get high and stay high. Rising cor-tisol levels result in severe hot flashes, no matter where your estrogen levels are. This may be because increased cortisol raises the body's core temperature and the body kicks off a hot flash to expel the ad-ditional heat. Cortisol thwarts insulin, so when cortisol is chronically high, you are essentially in a state of insulin resistance. We now know that's bad news when it comes to hot flashes.

Lowering cortisol and other stress hormones is one of the most ef-fective options for the relief of hot flashes out there.

Sluggish Liver

One of the liver's main jobs is to regulate blood sugar levels. A slug-gish liver is unable to do so, contributing to fluctuating or chroni-cally high levels of glucose. Your liver is Detoxification Central, in charge of breaking down toxins and used-up hormones such as es-trogen and preparing them for removal from the body. If these tox-ins and estrogens aren't handled properly, they can end up back in your bloodstream. This raises your body's overall toxic load and contributes to estrogen dominance, two highly inflammatory states that make you more susceptible to hot flashes.

What You Can Do to Relieve Hot Flashes and Night Sweats

Don't despair! The following essential oil blends, supplements, herbs, and self-care rituals are specifically designed to lessen the severity and frequency of hot flashes. Use these in concert with the Hormone Makeover Program in Part III to stabilize hormone levels, manage stress, reduce inflammation, and promote insulin sensitivity. Also turn to the chapters on stress and digestive issues for more help targeting those root causes.

If you've tried the natural approach and still need more assistance, check out the additional options for hot flashes at the end of this chapter. Always work with your functional healthcare provider to find the best way forward for you and your unique situation.

Each of the oils that I recommend below has been tested by thousands of women, so I know they provide hormonal support and either cooling relief (Peppermint and Clary Sage) or stress reduction (Lavender, Geranium, and Bergamot). Peppermint will always be my top oil for cooling relief due to its menthol content, so make that be the first oil in your arsenal against hot flashes. Any mint oil will provide a cooling sensation, so feel free to try Spearmint anywhere Peppermint is recommended in the recipes.

Top 5 Essential Oils for Hot Flash Relief

1. Peppermint
2. Clary Sage
3. Geranium
4. Bergamot
5. Lavender

Essential Oil Blends

Body Sprays

Hot Flash Spritz

7 drops Clary Sage essential oil
7 drops Peppermint essential oil
5 drops Geranium essential oil
Witch hazel

Spritz on the back of your neck, décolletage, and other areas where the sweats threaten during hot moments. Use as needed.

Rollerball Blends

Cool Down Rollerball Blend

10 drops Clary Sage essential oil
10 drops Peppermint essential oil
5 drops Geranium essential oil
Carrier oil of choice

Roll behind your ears, on the back of your neck, and on wrists and ankles.

Superwoman Rollerball Blend

12 drops Clary Sage essential oil
10 drops Lavender essential oil
5 drops Geranium essential oil
5 drops Cedarwood essential oil
4 drops Ylang Ylang essential oil
Carrier oil of choice

Roll on pulse points, especially wrists and behind ears.

Stress Balancing Rollerball Blend

10 drops Lavender essential oil
5 drops Geranium essential oil

5 drops Bergamot essential oil
4 drops Wild Orange essential oil
Carrier oil of choice

Apply to pulse points and bottoms of feet.

Hot Flash Support Supplements and Herbal Remedies

High-quality supplements can remedy the root causes behind your discomfort and help you find the relief you so desperately desire. In addition to the supplements I recommend as part of the 21-Day Hormone Makeover Program (page 257), consider adding the following.

Supplements

MAGNESIUM OXIDE (400–600 MG/DAY)

There are many different types of magnesium, and they each benefit your body in different ways. Magnesium oxide has been found to relieve hot flashes and enhance your ability to sleep without waking up in a sweat. It is a great short-term supplement to treat your hot flashes, but magnesium bis-glycinate is better for sustainably increasing your magnesium levels.

MYO-INOSITOL (500 MG/DAY)

Myo-inositol plays an important role in insulin regulation and reproductive health. Since insulin resistance is a key contributor to hot flashes, taking myo-inositol can help your cells become sensitive to insulin and relieve your discomfort.

BERBERINE (900–2,000 MG/DAY)

Berberine is a naturally occurring chemical derived from plants found to combat insulin resistance. It also prevents oxidation that damages your cells and cuts through inflammation to help alleviate the symptoms you are facing.

ESSENTIALLY WHOLE® HORMONE BALANCE

Hormone Balance contains an ideal blend of herbs, minerals, and nutrients to show your body the love it needs to achieve stable hormones and includes ingredients recognized for their ability to reduce hot flashes such as black cohosh, chaste tree, and DIM.

VITAMIN E

Vitamin E is an antioxidant with many health benefits, including the ability to help reduce hot flashes. A small 2007 study showed that consuming 400 IU of vitamin E every day helped reduce the severity, duration, and occurrence of hot flashes.

Herbs

RHUBARB (4 MG/DAY)

Rhubarb extract (sold as rhaponticin in the U.S.) has been used for decades in Europe to treat menopausal symptoms, including hot flashes. Your body processes it in a similar way to estrogen, so it can ease your transition without the harsh side effects of hormone replacement.

MACA (6-9 GRAMS/DAY)

Maca, a tuber native to Peru, is the staple source of protein and fiber in Andean diets. It is a powerful adaptogen that has been found to restore balance to your body and alleviate menopause discomforts, including hot flashes and night sweats. I recommend adding a scoop to your green smoothie in the morning for added energy, focus, and mood-boosting benefits.

ASHWAGANDHA (300–500 MG/DAY)

Ashwagandha is an adaptogenic herbal supplement found to safely alleviate many menopausal complaints, particularly hot flashes and night sweats.

Note: Some people with nightshade sensitivities react negatively to ashwagandha. Take this into account before you decide to give it a try!

VITEX/CHASTE TREE/CHASTEBERRY (150–250 MG/DAY)

Vitex, also known as chaste tree or chasteberry, is a well-recognized solution to balancing your hormones and is particularly helpful for relieving hot flashes and night sweats.

Dr. Mariza's Hormone-Loving Rituals and Protocols

Until you have stress under control, you will be harassed by the symptoms of hormone imbalance, including hot flashes and night sweats. Follow the stress-releasing Hormone-Loving Rituals and Protocols on page 87 plus the following.

Phytoestrogen Boost Routine

Phytoestrogens, natural estrogen-like hormones found in soy, flaxseeds, whole grains, fruits, and vegetables, can help balance estrogen levels and alleviate the nasty symptoms caused by an estrogenic imbalance such as hot flashes. In fact, adding 45–160 mg of phytoestrogens to your diet each day in the form of fruits, vegetables, or other superfoods such as flaxseeds can protect your body against certain cancers (including breast and colon) while balancing your estrogen levels. So, don't shy away from eating that soy unless you have specific recommendations from your healthcare provider. Its protective effects may greatly help to balance your overall estrogen levels and dial down those hot flashes.

Orgasmic Power

Yes! Did you know that some research suggests orgasm can help to reduce hot flashes? When you look at the physiological process of orgasm, it makes a lot of sense. You see, when a woman orgasms, it raises her estradiol levels, counteracting the low levels of estrogen that could lead to hot flashes. And increased pleasure means more oxytocin flowing through our veins, that feel-good hormone that we all need from intimate connection. In addition, oxytocin works with estrogen to eliminate high levels of cortisol in the body, the main hormone caused by stress.

All this means one thing: Sex does a body good! Stress-relieving, hormone-pumping orgasms could fix those pesky hot sweats.

Ginseng Tea Time Ritual

As a preventive measure, I recommend drinking a glass of red ginseng tea, which has been found to reduce hot flashes. In addition, you can also supplement by taking 3 g per day of red ginseng to support menopausal metabolism and cardiovascular function.

Additional Treatment Options for Hot Flashes

If you've tried natural options and your hot flashes and night sweats remain unmanageable, bioidentical hormones are another effective option to consider. Here's the deal: Hormone therapy has been shown to be the most effective therapy for hot flashes. But it's no magic bullet, remember? I always recommend talking with your trusted healthcare provider about any risks associated with your health history to create a plan that feels aligned with your health goals.

Bioidentical Estrogen

"Estrogen window" is the term to describe the period of time when using bioidentical estrogen can be beneficial in relieving menopausal symptoms, and the associated risks are more minimal. The estrogen window lasts for around five years, starting when a woman begins menopause, or slightly before.

It is important to note that women beginning estrogen *after* the estrogen window closes may increase their risk for breast cancer, osteoporosis, heart disease, and dementia. Please know these risks before making an informed decision with your trusted healthcare provider.

Bioidentical Progesterone

If estrogen is not a safe option for you, over-the-counter 2 percent natural progesterone has worked for women in perimenopause and menopause, and it's easy to use at home. Twenty mg ($^1/_4$ teaspoon applied to the hands, thighs, stomach area) once per day may provide relief from hot flashes. When asking your doctor for natural oral progesterone to manage menopause symptoms, refer to the pharmaceutical brand name: prometrium. Then your doctor knows exactly what you are asking for and will not accidentally prescribe a synthetic progesterone like progestin.

Chapter 7

Low Energy and Fatigue

Nicole, age fifty-five, came to me feeling depleted when she woke up and throughout the day. During our first conversation she shared the following: "Is this what fifty is supposed to feel like? I am tired and I can't escape this fog I am in each morning. It takes sheer willpower to get out of bed and get to work to teach each day. I want to crawl back into bed and sleep more. I have stopped working out because it exhausts me and sugar cravings get the best of me every time I walk into the teachers' lounge. I've put on seven pounds over the last three months. What can I do to fix this?"

Nicole presented with low cortisol levels in the morning, afternoon, and evening, chronic fatigue, and poor diet.

My recommendations were as follows:

- Six daily supplements: a multivitamin, 4,000 IU vitamin D, 400 mg magnesium glycinate, methylated B vitamins, 250 mg choline with inositol, and 2,000 mg omega-3 fatty acids to increase cellular energy and boost metabolic pathways.
- The 21-Day Hormone Makeover Meal Plan to reset eating habits and support healthy stress hormone changes.
- For afternoon slumps incorporate Instant Motivation Rollerball Blend (page 132) every hour, or diffuse energizing essential oils such as the Fatigue Zapper Diffuser Blend (page 131).

- Peppermint and Tangerine essential oils in the afternoon to reduce sugar cravings and boost energy.
- A 30-minute self-care Morning Ritual consisting of inhaling the Instant Motivation Rollerball Blend, gratitude journaling, a five-minute meditation, and a green smoothie.
- 20-minute nature walks 4–5 times a week during lunch breaks.

Four weeks later, a couple of days after completing the 21-Day Program, Nicole shared her results with me: "My extra weight is gone! Your program worked for me and I am feeling like a different person than the woman I was twenty-five days ago. The supplements really helped during the first two weeks of the program, and I continued to take them at breakfast and dinner. I do not need willpower to get out of bed to go teach my students, but I have more to go to completely restore my energy levels in the afternoon. In the meantime, the oil blends are really helping, especially as a distraction for not eating the treats in the teachers' room. I am loving the morning time to myself. The rituals are easy for me and I actually enjoy the smoothie and shakes. I am taking one for lunch, too, to make my life easier. I am continuing the program for breakfast and lunch and made a couple changes to dinner because overall, I am feeling less inflamed and more energized."

What's Going On

The most common phrases I hear from women, including myself at times, are "I'm tired," "I'm burned out," or "I just need a little more energy to get through my day."

And this fatigue is way more than tiredness from a rough week or a few late nights. It's a persistent bone-deep exhaustion that leaves you feeling weak and worn out physically, mentally, and emotionally, significantly impairing your daily function and quality of life. No amount of sleep—if you can get to sleep—leaves you refreshed or invigorated. You may be experiencing sleepiness, loss of appetite, digestive issues, frequent colds and other illnesses due to a weakened immune system, difficulty concentrating, slow reflexes, forgetfulness, depression, anxiety, irritability, and moodiness.

Why It's Happening

If your hormones are out of harmony, your energy levels will suffer. Energy drinks, sugar, and coffee can't power you through this fatigue, and trust me, those part-time solutions are only compounding other root cause issues in your body. Plus, so many hormonal imbalances disrupt your sleep, only adding to your misery. Here are the most likely hormone imbalances sapping your get-up-and-go.

Estrogen Dominance

Often referred to as the "feel-good hormone," progesterone is a natural antidepressant that promotes calm, tranquillity, and sleep. Low levels or an insufficient amount to balance out the effects of estrogen may make it difficult for you to relax and get enough quality rest and contributes to irritability, anxiety, depression, and brain fog.

Research also suggests that progesterone and estrogen may protect women against sleep apnea and other kinds of sleep-disordered breathing in which breathing briefly and repeatedly stops and starts throughout the night, causing fragmented sleep. The reduction of estrogen and progesterone that naturally occurs in menopause significantly reduces that benefit. The prevalence of sleep-disordered breathing in women doubles after menopause.

Low Testosterone

Fatigue, sluggishness, and muscle weakness are linked to low testosterone in women. Testosterone does more than help us maintain a healthy sex drive. It influences mood and energy levels, fostering motivation and emotional stamina, and supports strong, healthy bones and joints. A deficiency will put a damper on your total energy level. Testosterone also impacts levels of dopamine and serotonin, two neurotransmitters responsible for regulating mood and how vital we feel.

Thyroid Hormone Imbalance

Fatigue is the number one symptom for thyroid disorders, and was my first symptom of low thyroid function. I didn't catch it for almost two years because I thought it was just stress, and allowed myself to accept it as my normal. Fatigue isn't normal, especially bone-crushing fatigue. It's always worth getting your thyroid checked if your fatigue persists.

The thyroid regulates how your body uses energy, so an under- or overactive thyroid can leave you feeling drained and listless. Most women in perimenopause and menopause struggle with low thyroid function, or hypothyroidism. Without enough thyroid hormone, your whole body slows down. In hyperthyroidism, an overactive thyroid pumps out too much thyroid hormone, speeding your metabolism. The stress this puts on your body and metabolism makes it tough to sleep and, ultimately, depletes your body, causing fatigue.

Too Much Cortisol/HPA Axis Dysfunction

As we know, chronic stress triggers the adrenals to release increasing amounts of cortisol. A short burst of cortisol gives us the energy we need to survive an imminent threat, but over time, excess cortisol exhausts our body by upregulating our HPA axis, aka our stress response system. Now, instead of feeling fueled up and hard-charging, we're exhausted. In addition, cortisol's natural daily rhythm has been disrupted, making it tough for us to fall asleep and compounding our fatigue.

This is why it's best to limit caffeine. That cup of Earl Grey, piece of chocolate, or shot of espresso revs the adrenals to release cortisol. Keep in mind, it can take about six hours for the stimulant effects of caffeine to reduce by half, so that midafternoon jolt may be what's keeping you up at night.

Insulin Resistance

The standard American diet high in simple sugars and processed foods—bread, pasta, rice, potatoes, and sweetened beverages—has been shown to cause feelings of chronic sleepiness, daytime fatigue, poorer sleep, and slower cognitive performance. Eating a meal loaded with these foods immediately raises blood sugar levels. Sure, you'll feel a burst of energy as a surge of insulin quickly gets to work firing up your cells, but once its work is done and blood sugar levels plummet, the crash will inevitably follow. This yo-yo response contributes to fatigue and, if it happens regularly, will lead to insulin resistance, when your cells don't respond to insulin anymore and glucose can't enter. It's simple: Cells that can't get the energy they need from glucose stop functioning at peak capacity. Plus, the additional glucose circulating in your system causes your blood to flow less well, as if there were sugar in your car's gas tank, slowing you down.

Stress/Rushing Woman's Syndrome

I've watched my patients and friends go from stressed out to burned out due to endless, unrelenting chronic stress. Stress and fatigue create a vicious downward spiral, as one fuels the other in a whirlwind of destruction. Worries, anxiety, and depression from stress can make it difficult to get to sleep and stay that way through the night, leaving you feeling tired all the time. In addition, chronic stress can fuel chronic pain, making it even more difficult to rest and promoting even more intense and lasting stress. The severe hit your immune system takes from chronic stress makes you vulnerable to infections and sickness, another serious drain on your energy reserves.

We can't avoid stress; it's a part of life to a certain degree. But the way we handle stress may impact how tired we feel. In one study, participants who avoided dealing with stress experienced the greatest level of fatigue. This is why it is so important to value self-care in your life.

Poor or Low-Quality Sleep

The right amount of good-quality sleep leaves you feeling refreshed and restored for a reason. During the night over the course of several uninterrupted hours of sleep, your brain and body recharge, repairing muscle, storing memories, and releasing hormones that regulate growth and appetite. If you're not getting enough sleep—and many of us aren't—I probably don't have to tell you that you'll feel miserable and exhausted.

According to the National Sleep Foundation, adults ages twenty-six to sixty-four need seven to nine hours of sleep, while adults sixty-five years and older need slightly less—seven to eight hours. While we should all aim for enough sleep, it's the quality of that sleep that matters. If you take longer than thirty minutes to fall asleep, wake up more than once during the night and struggle to fall back to sleep, and have to drag yourself out of bed the next morning, your sleep quality needs attention.

Mitochondrial Dysfunction

Mitochondria are the "energy powerhouses" of the body. Several thousand of them are in nearly every cell, and their role is to turn the raw material of the food we eat into the energy our body needs to function. When your mitochondria are in tip-top condition, your cells are able to produce enough energy to keep you humming. But if the mitochondria become damaged or stop functioning, we're starved of fuel at the cellular level. You're literally trying to run on an empty tank.

Mitochondria don't become dysfunctional on their own:

- **Poor diet**. Energy production relies on certain vitamins and minerals, especially B vitamins. Without them, the necessary chemical reactions can't occur and the process stalls.
- **Lack of movement.** Muscles contain the most mitochondria, since they need the most energy for movement and exercise.

The more we move and demand of our mitochondria, the more energy they produce and the more mitochondria the muscle cells produce, making tasks easier. When we're sedentary, we have fewer mitochondria, so less available energy, and the ones we do have are quickly zapped.

- **Inflammation.** Chronic inflammation causes mitochondria to switch, Jekyll and Hyde like from energy generators to toxin-producing factories, promoting more inflammation.
- **Circadian rhythm dysfunction.** Mitochondria do their work in sync with our circadian rhythm, our twenty-four-hour internal clock. If we're out of sync, mitochondria function is impaired and energy declines.

Too Little or Too Much Activity

The heart is a muscle and it atrophies with lack of exertion. A weak heart, pumping less blood with each beat, means low energy. "Saving" your energy for later by taking the elevator instead of the stairs isn't a good plan. Being active goes a long way toward amping up energy. A University of Georgia study showed that sedentary people who regularly complained of fatigue increased their energy levels by 20 percent and decreased their fatigue by 65 percent by engaging in regular low-intensity exercise. Exercise can also lead to more high-quality sleep, leaving you alert and refreshed, especially in adults over sixty-five. Plus, the endorphins released during exercise are a natural mood and energy booster.

Too much of a good thing, in this case exercise, can be a bad thing. Too much vigorous, high-intensity exercise that pushes your body to the limit is a form of stress. And when your body is stressed, it's primed for fight or flight—not the restorative sleep your body needs to repair and revitalize. Movement is designed to regenerate you, not deplete you. If pushing yourself as hard as you can for an hour several times a week is leaving you tired—and you're not seeing the hoped-for results—it's time to reset your workout routine.

When Fatigue Becomes Chronic

Chronic fatigue syndrome (CFS), also known as myalgic encephalomyelitis (ME), or by both names as ME/CFS, plagues many people with extreme fatigue yet seemingly no underlying medical condition or explanation. Rest rarely helps and symptoms are exacerbated by mental or physical exertion.

Anyone can get ME/CFS, but it is most common in people between forty and sixty years old, and women are two to four times more likely than men to develop ME/CFS. One study suggests a potential link between ME/CFS and early menopause, especially hysterectomy-related menopause, but more research needs to be done to understand the possible connection.

Since there is no one test for ME/CFS, a diagnosis rests on working with your trusted healthcare provider to eliminate all other potential sources of your fatigue. We don't yet know the cause of ME/CFS, so the best we can do is treat the symptoms. In my practice, I've found that addressing the most common root causes underlying hormone imbalance and building a healthy foundation of good diet, exercise, and adequate sleep, while reducing stress and supporting the body with essential oils, can greatly influence the effects of ME/CFS. The Hormone Makeover Program in Part III can help you get on the right track once your healthcare provider has signed off on it.

What You Can Do to Increase Energy and Fight Fatigue

It's hard to make lifestyle changes to promote healthy hormone function when you are wiped out, tired, and miserable. Fortunately, if you struggle with fatigue, the following essential oil blends, supplements, herbs, and self-care rituals are specifically designed to support sustainable energy. Use these in concert with the Hormone Makeover Program in Part III and turn to the chapters on stress and sleep, if you suspect those are at the root of your fatigue.

Top 5 Essential Oils to Increase Energy and Fight Fatigue

1. Citrus Essential Oils
   - *Bergamot*
   - *Lemon*
   - *Lime*
   - *Tangerine*
   - *Wild Orange*
2. Peppermint
3. Rosemary
4. Eucalyptus
5. Basil

Essential Oil Blends

Diffuser Blends

Fatigue Zapper Diffuser Blend

3 drops Eucalyptus essential oil
3 drops Peppermint essential oil

Energy Boost Diffuser Blend

2 drops Wild Orange essential oil (or your favorite Citrus)
2 drops Peppermint essential oil

Focused Energy Diffuser Blend

3 drops Rosemary essential oil
2 drops Peppermint essential oil
I drop Basil essential oil

Personal Inhaler Blends

Exercise-Enhancing Inhaler Blend

4 drops Peppermint essential oil

4 drops Eucalyptus essential oil

2 drops Rosemary essential oil

2 drops Lavender essential oil

2 drops Lemon (or favorite Citrus) essential oil

Morning Energy Inhaler Blend

5 drops Rosemary essential oil

5 drops Peppermint essential oil

5 drops Wild Orange (or your favorite Citrus) essential oil

Aromatic Spray

Energize a Room Spray

10 drops Peppermint essential oil

10 drops Eucalyptus essential oil

8 drops Bergamot essential oil

Distilled water or witch hazel

Rollerball Blends

Energy Restored Rollerball Blend

10 drops Peppermint essential oil

10 drops Wild Orange essential oil

Carrier oil of choice

Apply to pulse points, especially behind the ears, throughout the day as needed.

Instant Motivation Rollerball Blend

6 drops Peppermint essential oil

6 drops Wild Orange (or your favorite Citrus) essential oil

4 drops Frankincense essential oil (or 6 drops Bergamot essential oil)

2 drops Basil essential oil

2 drops Rosemary essential oil

Carrier oil of choice

Apply to pulse points, especially behind the ears and on wrists, throughout the day.

Wake Up Energized Rollerball Blend

8 drops Spearmint essential oil

8 drops Eucalyptus essential oil

4 drops Lavender essential oil

4 drops Lemon essential oil

Carrier oil of choice

Apply to pulse points, especially behind the ears, to fuel and energize your workout.

Morning Abundance Rollerball Blend

7 drops Peppermint essential oil

7 drops Wild Orange essential oil

6 drops Frankincense essential oil (optional)

2 drops Basil essential oil

Carrier oil of choice

Apply to pulse points, especially behind the ears and on wrists and ankles.

Energy-Supporting Supplements and Herbal Remedies

Supplements are an efficient way to get your cells the energy they need without the jittery, crashing feeling that follows a few hours after that caffeine or sugar fix. Instead of waiting for fatigue to hit, developing a healthy energy-boosting supplement routine can promote your overall health in a way that prevents you from becoming drained in the first place. In addition to the supplements I recommend as part of the 21-Day Makeover Plan (page 272), here are a few of my favorites.

Supplements

VITAMIN D (4,000–5,000 IU/DAY)

This "sunshine" vitamin actually acts more like a hormone in your body than a vitamin. Every cell in your body has a receptor for vitamin D, and most of us are deficient thanks to being inside most of the time and wearing sunscreen when we do venture out.

Getting enough vitamin D by supplementing with vitamin D3 can help reduce insulin resistance and support healthy cell function to get the most energy from the food you eat. Not only that, most women who take vitamin D report significant changes in their fatigue and also their mood thanks to its role in increasing dopamine and serotonin levels.

ADRENAL LOVE BY ESSENTIALLY WHOLE®

Formulated with specific vitamins and adaptogenic herbs, such as vitamin C, ashwagandha, and rhodiola, Adrenal Love provides HPA axis regulation that will boost your energy, calm your overactive stress responses, and stabilize your blood sugar levels.

Note: Ashwagandha is in the nightshade family, so use caution if you are sensitive to them.

IRON (30–50 MG/DAY)

Low iron leaves your cells lacking oxygen, leaving you feeling weak and fatigued. Getting enough iron is one of the best ways to safeguard yourself against feelings of exhaustion.

MITOCHONDRIAL ESSENTIAL COFACTORS

As the powerhouses of your cells, mitochondria can use a little help as you enter menopause to keep your cells energized and working their best. Here are a few cofactors, or helpers, that you can supplement with (and combine to get the best results):

Alpha-lipoic acid (300–600 mg/day) helps turn the food you eat into energy, keeps blood sugar low, and reduces inflammation that can slow your cells down. This compound can work in every cell of your body to help them stay energized and clear of substances that slow them down!

Acetyl-L-carnitine (630-2,500 mg/day) supplements improve energy levels, particularly in your muscles, so this is a great one to use if exercising is part of your daily routine. It can also promote feel-good brain chemicals to help beat mental fatigue at the root.

Coenzyme Q10 (50–100 mg/day) is essential for your cells to have the energy they need to thrive. It's common for your natural levels to decline as you approach menopause, so supplementing with CoQ10 is a great way to keep your mitochondria thriving!

Herbs

HOLY BASIL (1,100–2,900 MG/DAY)

Holy basil is a powerhouse supplement to aid your energy naturally, lessening physical and psychological stress, improving sleep, normalizing blood sugar levels, and reducing feelings of exhaustion.

ASHWAGANDHA (300–500 MG/DAY) AND RHODIOLA (START AT 50 MG/DAY AND STEADILY INCREASE UNTIL YOU ACHIEVE DESIRED RESULTS, BUT DO NOT EXCEED 680 MG/DAY)

These two adaptogens work to powerfully relieve your feelings of mental and physical fatigue. With anti-inflammatory, anti-stress, and hormone/nervous system–supporting properties, ashwagandha and rhodiola make my top list of energy supplements.

Note: If you're sensitive to nightshades, these can be a trigger for some people. So just beware before you start implementing them into your routine!

MACA (1,500–3,000 MG/DAY)

Maca supports healthy hormone balance and reduces your feelings of stress and anxiety in order to make you feel more energized.

ROYAL JELLY (50–300 MG/DAY)

Royal jelly is the substance produced by honeybees to feed the queen and her young. Rich in B vitamins and with powerful anti-inflammatory properties, royal jelly treats many of the root causes that could be driving your exhaustion. It is a great supplement to work into your routine if you struggle with blood sugar and insulin imbalances. It has also been found to relieve anxiety that could be making you feel more tired.

Dr. Mariza's Hormone-Loving Rituals and Protocols

A regular morning routine is my secret for beginning each day feeling rejuvenated and energized. Follow the Morning Ritual suggestions on page 87 and then work the energy-boosting power of essential oils throughout the day. Find the diffuser recipe or rollerball blend that delivers that instant energy boost and keep it with you at all times.

Nature Walk Ritual

Time spent outdoors will also boost your energy levels and reinvigorate your spirit. Find a regular time of day—maybe during your midafternoon slump time—to take a brisk walk. Even ten minutes will help, but aim for a good thirty minutes to boost those vitamin D levels and get your body rebalanced. And if you aren't able to get enough natural sunlight, try light therapy.

Chapter 8

Mood Swings, Anxiety, and Depression

Teresa had experienced anxiety for most of her life. When I met her, she was fifty and her anxiety was at an all-time high. Teresa shared with me that her anxiety would come out of nowhere and it felt like a tightness in her chest, shoulders, and neck. She felt isolated and anxious at work and it was causing her to miss project meetings. When I asked her about the frequency, she said, "The feeling can really vary for me. Some days it feels debilitating and other days I can manage it. I started to really notice everything change about three months ago when my periods got really erratic and my flow became very heavy. I'm also experiencing occasional migraines. It all feels so sudden, but I am sure I am getting closer to menopause. My mom didn't experience menopause until she was fifty-two. Is there anything natural that I can do? I really don't want to take medications, but I also can't continue like this much longer without relief."

Teresa was experiencing perimenopause hormone fluctuation, symptoms of estrogen dominance and anxiousness.

My recommendations were as follows:

- Six daily supplements: 1,000 mg vitamin C, 2,000 mg omega-3 fatty acids, 450 mg St. John's Wort, 4 capsules Essentially

Whole® Hormone Balance, 400 mg magnesium glycinate, 1–2 chewable tablets Essentially Whole® Calm & Restore to support mood, hormone levels, and increase energy.

- Focus on gut- and liver-loving foods by making morning green smoothies and salads for lunch from the 21-Day Program.
- Drink holy basil and matcha green tea in the afternoon. L-theanine reduces stress and feelings of anxiousness.
- Schedule dates with girlfriends throughout the weekend and in the evenings.
- Nature walks for 30 minutes, 4–5 times a week during lunch, to boost happy neurotransmitters and increase energy.
- For feeling of anxiousness at work, apply the Soothe Anxious Feelings Rollerball Blend (page 149) and use the Deep Breathing ritual (page 88), or 5-minute meditation.
- 20-minute Morning Ritual: Daily Self-Care Journal (page 266), diffuse happy citrus oils, and write out self-love affirmations.

A little more than three weeks later Teresa updated me on how she was doing; I could tell from her voice that she was feeling happier and relaxed. "I started with the easiest things first and solutions that would immediately help me when my anxiety got bad at work. The breath work and essential oil blend worked better than I imagined. I have been using the breath technique every day, even on days when I don't feel anxious. I want my body to get used to feeling calm. I also love my morning rituals. I never had an actual ritual before, and I noticed that they really ease my mind for the rest of my day. There are probably other benefits that I haven't noticed yet. Lastly, the supplements and diet recommendations have helped a lot with my heavy bleeding, mood swings, and bloating. I know they have helped my anxiety, too, but it's harder to measure. I am going to continue many of the recommendations, especially the ones that directly help my anxiety. I feel so much better and don't plan to revert back."

What's Going On

You're living on top of the world one minute and close to tears the next, racked by worried thoughts that just won't quit, or stuck under a dark cloud you can't seem to shake. Many women report an increase in mood swings, anxiety, and depression during perimenopause and menopause, so know you're not alone. It's natural to experience emotional highs and lows, but this time of life is especially challenging for many reasons, and hormonal changes are only a part of the story.

Perimenopause and menopause are natural times of transition. Your body and life are changing in ways you may not always want or welcome, which can cause a grieving process. The winding down or end of your fertility may be bittersweet or prompt you to start thinking more about your purpose and goals. Your children may have left the nest and your circle of friends might not be as tight as it once was, leaving you feeling more lonely or isolated. It's okay if you struggle. It's okay to feel sad, angry, tense, or uncertain about the next stage of your life. It's good to acknowledge what you are feeling and the fears you may be facing. This is especially important if you are more vulnerable to anxiety and depression.

This can be a difficult time. But it doesn't have to be. There are things you can do to help move forward with power and grace. In most cases, changes in mood are perfectly normal bumps in the road that will improve by making choices that support hormone balance. The turnaround I saw in my mother's mood once she committed to the Hormone Makeover Program was nothing short of amazing. Her depression and listlessness lifted and her energy restored. And yours can, too.

Mood Swings. These have rocked my world for years—just ask my husband! Happy one minute, down in the dumps the next. So angry I'm seeing red and then laughing moments later. Cheery and upbeat on Monday, crabby and negative on Tuesday. Riding these highs and lows left me feeling tired, frustrated, and out of control. Mood swings are one of the most common symptoms of perimenopause, with up to

70 percent of women describing irritability, being less tolerant and more easily annoyed, as their biggest emotional issue during this time.

Anxiety. Anxiety—feelings of tension, nervousness, and worry—threatens our outlook on life, causing many of us to wake up troubled and uneasy and tread water throughout the day just to keep ourselves above the surface. People with anxiety may deal with panic attacks or withdraw from society to cope. Anxiety can become the most crippling manifestation of stress there is, and it's very common. More than half of women aged forty to fifty-five report occasional anxiety, and a quarter report frequent bouts of day-ruining anxiety, with lightheadedness, nausea, diarrhea, and a frequent need to pee as the most common symptoms. Plus, chronic anxiety can increase your risk for heart disease and gastrointestinal conditions.

Depression. Depression is one of those not-so-pleasant symptoms of perimenopause and menopause that we don't like to talk about. Everyone is always telling us to think positive and look on the bright side. We're worried that no one wants to hear how we really feel, so we put on our happy face and hide the fact that we've been struggling for some time now with sadness, hopelessness, and apathy. Maybe you feel stuck in an unsatisfying job, a dead-end relationship, or a cycle of mounting debt. You may have problems sleeping and overeating or loss of appetite. If this sounds like you, you're not in this alone. A CDC study found that about one out of ten women in the United States experience symptoms of depression, with an increase to one out of every five women as they move through menopause. And not only does depression have the potential to rob you of the joy of life and prevent you from making positive changes, but people with depression are also more likely to have inflammatory conditions or autoimmune disorders and coronary artery disease.

If you're experiencing symptoms of anxiety or depression, you may be considering a trip to your trusted healthcare provider to discuss the possibility of anti-anxiety or antidepressant medication. Before you do this, let me encourage you to try a more holistic approach first. You see, prescription drugs don't really fix the underlying issue.

They're sort of a stopgap solution. For starters, they don't address the underlying hormonal changes that are most likely the root cause of your anxiety or depression. Secondly, it has been estimated that a significant percentage of individuals on antidepressants don't actually see any marked improvement of their symptoms. Yikes! All that money for nothing. Thirdly, as you know, all drugs have potential side effects. Why risk developing side effects such as nausea, insomnia, agitation, weight gain, sexual dysfunction, and cardiovascular events if there is a natural solution?

Of course, there is no magic bullet to heal emotional distress. Essential oils cannot cure a mood disorder, but they support us on the journey. *A lot.* Especially if what we are dealing with isn't a mood disorder but rather a hormonal imbalance caused by the menopausal transition, chronic stress, gut issues, and/or lifestyle choices.

Clinical Depression and Anxiety

Please don't ignore or deny your symptoms. If they are interfering with your daily life and relationships, seek professional support.

Clinical depression, also known as major depression or major depressive disorder, is a constant sense of severe hopelessness and despair that makes it difficult for you to function day to day every day for at least two weeks.

Clinical anxiety refers to specific disorders involving overwhelming and disabling worry and fear that keep you from carrying on with your life normally. These include generalized anxiety disorder (GAD), panic disorder and panic attacks, agoraphobia, social anxiety disorder, selective mutism, separation anxiety, and specific phobias.

A trusted healthcare professional can work with your specific symptoms and root issues to ensure that you receive the care that you need. If your symptoms are severe and you need

Why It's Happening

Healthy hormonal balance keeps our emotions and moods balanced, too. The hormone shifts during perimenopause and menopause have a direct influence on how we feel and contribute to mood swings, anxiety, and depression. These are some of the most common hormonal imbalances and root causes contributing to your emotional well-being.

Wild Hormone Fluctuations

All reproductive hormones, including progesterone, estrogen, and testosterone, impact mood, focus, and cognitive function, as receptor sites for these hormones are found throughout the central nervous system and brain. In perimenopause, these hormones are riding a roller coaster, which means your brain is riding a roller coaster, too, resulting in potentially erratic feelings of anger, impatience, and sadness. Estrogen is also related to the production of serotonin, the "happy" hormone and neurotransmitter that plays an important role in regulating mood. Fluctuating estrogen and serotonin leads to mood swings. In menopause, hormone levels tend to stabilize so you're not dealing with erratic shifts anymore, but you are dealing with low levels of these hormones, linked to irritability, anxiety, and difficulty concentrating.

Low Estrogen

Your brain relies on estrogen to function optimally, so lower levels may mean it's not getting as much as it needs. Estrogen helps to regulate several mood-boosting hormones, such as serotonin, norepinephrine, and dopamine, which have a profound effect on your mood and sense of well-being. Low levels of estrogen are linked to depression, anxiety, irritability, insomnia, fatigue, and a decreased sense of pleasure in life. A decrease in estrogen can also cause brain fog, and there's nothing like a fuzzy brain to kick off frustration, anxiety, and a blue mood.

Low Progesterone

Progesterone is the first hormone to decline in perimenopause and settles at a much lower level in menopausal women than in women of reproductive age. While estrogen is important for maintaining healthy emotional balance, progesterone is equally important for maintaining your equilibrium. A calming hormone at optimal levels, low progesterone may cause depression, anxiety, irritability, and insomnia.

Stress

Stress, especially chronic stress, does a number on our bodies and minds, capable of triggering mood swings, anxiety, and depression. After listening to thousands of women's experiences, I realized that feeling stressed out is the number one culprit for our mood issues, causing a cascade of hormonal imbalances and emotional distress.

As you know by now, chronic stress is a major factor in elevating cortisol levels. Left unchecked, high cortisol results in feelings of overwhelm and worry and is closely linked to depression. One study found that nearly 50 percent of severely depressed individuals have elevated cortisol levels. Compounding the problem, high cortisol throws off your estrogen, progesterone, and thyroid hormones, leading to dropping levels of serotonin and other neurotransmitters that keep your mood balanced. It also shuts down your digestive system and, since most serotonin is produced in the gut, your mood will seriously suffer. Lots of cortisol over long periods of time can lead to insulin resistance and a disruption in the way the brain responds to dopamine, a neurotransmitter involved in pleasure, reward, and motivation. This can sabotage your mood and lead to symptoms of anxiety and depression. Finally, chronic stress ramps up inflammation in the body, and several studies have found links between inflammation, depression, and anxiety.

Prioritizing self-care and other lifestyle changes to relieve your stress burden, now and long-term, is one of the most powerful ways to improve your emotional well-being. It can immediately make a difference in your life!

Trauma

Traumatic life events were found to be the biggest single cause of anxiety and depression, in a study by researchers at the University of Liverpool. And a new study suggests that women who suffered trauma during their teens, such as emotional abuse, parental separation or divorce, or living with someone with alcohol or substance addiction, have a greater risk of developing depression during perimenopause.

Do you ever find yourself making decisions from a place of past trauma? I do, but not intentionally. There are times when my twelve-year-old self is calling all the shots and I feel like I'm just along for the ride. And have you noticed that you never quite know when you are going to feel triggered? In fact, anything that gets us worked up and upset is probably pushing a trauma button, firing off patterns of past betrayal, shame, abandonment, and unworthiness. Until I properly dealt with my past trauma, I continued to unravel at a moment's notice when my stress levels were high. This became an important part of healing my body and mind, and I encourage you to address your past trauma and see how it may have affected your Health-Life Timeline (see page 37).

Lack of Sleep

Several nights of inadequate shut-eye can add to irritability, mood swings, anxiety, and depression. Disrupted sleep prevents you from getting enough quality REM sleep, the restorative sleep that supports learning, memory, and emotional health. It also upsets the balance of mood-enhancing neurotransmitters such as serotonin and dopamine. And, wouldn't you know, while lack of sleep can worsen mood, symptoms of anxiety and depression can contribute to sleep troubles. Getting good sleep during perimenopause and menopause can already seem like a very tall order, but the link is clear: Better sleep equals better mood.

Low Thyroid Function

Your thyroid has multiple roles in your body: controlling your metabolism, helping regulate your blood sugar, and helping control the release of stress hormones. A deficiency of thyroid hormones is linked to depression and anxiety. According to one study, about 45 percent of people with depression and 30 percent with anxiety also have Hashimoto's, an autoimmune condition that weakens the thyroid; and depression and anxiety were both significantly more common in those with Hashimoto's. Low thyroid function is very common in women during perimenopause and menopause and might be throwing off your mood. And I can personally speak to this through my Hashimoto's diagnosis. Getting to the root cause of my condition helped to regulate my mood, and I am a stronger woman because of it!

Gut Issues

With more nerve endings than even your spinal cord, the gut is responsible for producing many of the neurotransmitters associated with mood. In fact, it manufactures more than 90 percent of your "happy" hormone serotonin. Low serotonin can cause a variety of mood imbalances. With such a powerful impact on your emotions, it's more than fitting that the gut has been dubbed "the second brain." If your gut is irritated, your brain is going to hear about it.

The rest of your body will, too, as poor gut health kindles chronic inflammation, overwhelmingly linked to mood swings, anxiety, and depression. Markers of inflammation are elevated in people who suffer from depression compared to nondepressed ones.

Making sure your gut is working properly—lowering stress, reducing inflammatory foods, and supporting a healthy microbiome—will send the right signals to your brain, lower inflammation, and help resolve mood issues.

PMS and PMDD

If you have a history of intense PMS or PMDD, you're more likely to experience severe mood swings during perimenopause, from mild irritability and anxiety to full-blown depression, panic attacks, and severe rage. As your cycle becomes more irregular and your hormone fluctuations escalate, all of your PMS and PMDD symptoms, including cramps, headaches, tender breasts, bloating, and mood issues, will likely get worse, though their ferocity may change from month to month. My mother is a classic case, as her wild mood swings and anger escalated as she approached menopause. Don't ignore them! This does not need to be your "new normal."

A lifestyle reset promoting hormone balance, especially between estrogen and progesterone, will help. I know that when I've not done right by my body during the month, my PMS will bite me in the booty big-time. The better I take care of myself, the less my PMS symptoms will rock my world. It'll do wonders for you, too!

What You Can Do to Support Your Mood

One of the most researched areas of aromatherapy is the effect essential oils have on emotions and mood. They can't cure a mood disorder, but we know they can give you an edge on toning down your stress levels, promoting sleep, and providing the support we need to make lifestyle choices that promote a balanced mood. Through their primary constituents, essential oils can affect the body in three main ways: uplift and energize; calm and soothe; and ground and balance. Figuring out which essential oils work best for your individual body chemistry takes time. I recommend starting with one oil and trying it for several days. Be persistent and consistent. You may find all it takes is one whiff from the bottle of Peppermint essential oil to instantly lift your mood, but you may need to adorn your pulse points multiple times a day with Lavender to get the calming effect that you need. Listen to what your body is telling you.

Use these in concert with the Hormone Makeover Program in Part III to start feeling like yourself again. Also turn to the chapters on sleep, stress, hot flashes, and digestive issues for more help targeting those root causes.

Top 5 Essential Oils for Emotional Balance

1. Bergamot
2. Copaiba
3. Ylang Ylang
4. Lavender
5. Sandalwood

Essential Oil Blends

Diffuser Blends

Release Anxious Feelings Diffuser Blend

2 drops Sandalwood essential oil
2 drops Bergamot essential oil
1 drop Ylang Ylang essential oil
1 drop Patchouli essential oil

Tension Release Diffuser Blend

2 drops Geranium essential oil
2 drops Bergamot essential oil
2 drops Copaiba essential oil

Breathe and Release Diffuser Blend

3 drops Bergamot essential oil

2 drops Cedarwood essential oil

2 drops Spearmint essential oil

2 drops Lavender essential oil

Love Yourself Diffuser Blend

3 drops Bergamot essential oil

2 drops Sandalwood or Cedarwood essential oil

1 drop Ylang Ylang essential oil

Personal Inhaler Blends

Emotional Support Inhaler Blend

7 drops Wild Orange essential oil

4 drops Lavender essential oil

2 drops Copaiba essential oil

2 drops Ylang Ylang essential oil

Grounded Calm Inhaler Blend

4 drops Bergamot essential oil

4 drops Lavender essential oil

4 drops Frankincense essential oil

3 drops Cedarwood or Copaiba essential oil

Rollerball Blends

Soothe Anxious Feelings Rollerball Blend

8 drops Copaiba essential oil

6 drops Bergamot essential oil

3 drops Patchouli or Sandalwood essential oil

3 drops Ylang Ylang essential oil

Carrier oil of choice

Apply to pulse points and the back of your neck.

Emotional Release Rollerball Blend

6 drops Copaiba essential oil

6 drops Bergamot essential oil

5 drops Jasmine or Clary Sage essential oil

5 drops Ylang Ylang essential oil

Carrier oil of choice

Apply to pulse points and massage deeply into skin to promote emotional release.

Trauma Soothe Rollerball Blend

6 drops Clary Sage essential oil

5 drops Lavender essential oil

5 drops Sandalwood essential oil

5 drops Tangerine essential oil

2 drops Copaiba essential oil

Carrier oil of choice

Apply to pulse points and the back of your neck.

Mood-Supporting Supplements and Herbal Remedies

I'm going to say it again: Never ignore your symptoms. If you suspect clinical anxiety or depression, it is important that you seek out professional help immediately.

That being said, there are natural alternatives to antidepressants if your symptoms are on the milder side. There's even preliminary research that indicates some of these work as well—if not better—than their prescription counterparts! In addition to the supplements I recommend as part of the 21-Day Makeover Plan (page 272), here are some more of my go-to supplements and adaptogenic herbs to support mood stability.

Supplements

SAMe (S-ADENOSYL-L-METHIONINE) (600–1,200 MG/DAY)

SAMe is a naturally occurring molecule found in plants, bacteria, and humans that plays a vital role in converting the amino acids you get in your diet into key neurotransmitters such as serotonin, dopamine, and norepinephrine. Research shows that SAMe has powerful anti-depression effects when you ingest it. Because it helps boost levels of feel-good neurotransmitters, SAMe supplements are a safe way to combat mild depression, anxiety, and mood problems. Get the most power out of your SAMe supplement by pairing it with B-complex vitamins, essential counterparts for SAMe to be effective.

L-THEANINE (100–200 MG/DAY)

L-theanine is a great supplement to support the production of your brain's calming neurotransmitters to reduce feelings of stress, promote higher-quality sleep, and suppress anxious or racing thoughts.

Herbs

ST. JOHN'S WORT (300 MG THREE TIMES A DAY [900 MG DAILY])

St. John's Wort is a natural way to boost your body's serotonin levels, leading to increased positivity and mental calm to allow your mood to stabilize.

Please note that it can interact negatively with some prescriptions (especially ones designed for sleep or anxiety), so talk to your trusted healthcare provider before starting St. John's Wort if you take any other medications.

ASHWAGANDHA (300–500 MG/DAY)

Ashwagandha is a powerful herb that has the ability to regulate a stressed-out nervous system and calm your anxious mind. It is also a powerful anti-inflammatory agent, which can help resolve your mood instability from the root.

Note: Ashwagandha is a nightshade and can trigger reactions in people sensitive to them; use with caution.

RHODIOLA (START AT 50 MG/DAY AND STEADILY INCREASE UNTIL YOU ACHIEVE DESIRED RESULTS, BUT DO NOT EXCEED 680 MG/DAY)

Research indicates that rhodiola may have similar effects to prescription antidepressants, but without the adverse effects. While it can't replace stronger medications in every case, if you are facing mild or moderate symptoms of anxiety and depression and are wanting to avoid the risks associated with prescriptions, rhodiola is a great place to start.

SAFFRON (15 MG, TWICE PER DAY)

An effective, natural alternative to some depression treatments, saffron shows promise as a way to promote healthy mood stability. Preliminary research shows that it is just as effective as conventional drug treatments for depression, but without the side effects.

Dr. Mariza's Hormone-Loving Rituals and Protocols

My morning routine sets the tone for my day by setting me up with intention and positivity. Follow my Morning Ritual recommendations (page 87) and try the following.

"Is This Serving Me?" Ritual

One of the most important questions you can ask yourself about almost anything pertaining to your physical and emotional well-being is: "Is this serving me?" Take a moment and gut check with yourself. Is this event or task supporting your success, your happiness, your worth? If what you're doing isn't serving you, if it's causing you anxiety or worry, then it's worth reevaluating. Asking yourself this all-important question empowers you to say *no*—and make a change.

Here's how it works. You go out to dinner after work with some friends and everyone is ordering drinks. Take a moment and ask yourself: "Would a glass of wine serve me right now?" You get to decide if a glass of wine serves you, or if a sparkling water would support you more. It's not about feeling bad or shameful. It's about simply asking yourself what's right for you right now.

Overcome Overwhelm Ritual

Acknowledge that you hold power in your own life. Endless obligations and to-do lists may try to derail you, but ultimately *you* choose how to respond. When life starts to feel overwhelming, take a moment, pause, and begin to breathe deeply. Reach for your Emotional Release Rollerball Blend or Superwoman Rollerball Blend and roll it on your pulse points, inhaling in its scent. Remind yourself: "I am powerful. I am in control." Whenever overwhelm threatens to zap your power, take a moment and recharge with this ritual.

Chapter 9

Thyroid Issues

Kelley reached out to me after hearing that I had Hashimoto's thyroiditis. At age forty-nine, she had recently noticed symptoms of low thyroid function. She was experiencing symptoms of brain fog, fatigue, brittle hair, mild depression, constipation, and erratic, shorter periods. She explained: "It feels like someone placed a heavy veil over me. I am worn down and worn out. Initially, my doctors just told me I was going into menopause and that my symptoms were normal for my age. I went to another doctor because my best friend was diagnosed with thyroid issues and she had some of the same issues I am experiencing. I knew it was worth digging a bit more. My thyroid labs came back normal, except that my Free T4 was on the low end and my TPO antibodies were very high. That's when I knew I had Hashimoto's, but I must have caught it early enough. Now I am trying to figure out what I can do to feel better. I know that things slow down as we get older, but it can't be this bad. Is there anything I can do to at least increase my energy, brain function, and happiness?"

Kelley was experiencing low thyroid symptoms, Hashimoto's, elevated cortisol, and she was approaching menopause with wild hormone fluctuations.

My recommendations were as follows:

- Five daily supplements: methylated B vitamin complex, 400 mg magnesium glycinate, 2 capsules Essentially Whole® Thyroid

Support, 4,000 IU vitamin D, and 2,000 mg omega-3 fatty acids to support thyroid function, lower stress and inflammation, and increase energy.

- Gut supporting supplements: Digestive enzymes and probiotics
- The 21-Day Hormone Makeover Meal Plan to reset blood sugar levels, support liver and estrogen detoxification, and support healthy metabolic changes.
- Holy basil or decaffeinated tea in the morning and evening to reduce feelings of stress.
- 20-minute Morning Ritual: Daily Self-Care Journal (page 266) and Mindfulness Meditation.
- Five- to ten-minute meditations in the morning and afternoon with a mediation app (Headspace or Stop, Breathe & Think app).
- For daytime energy slumps use the Wake Up Energized Rollerball Blend (page 133).
- For stress, use the De-Stress Rollerball Blend (page 84) with Deep Breathing ritual (page 88).

Four weeks later Kelley reported her progress and was experiencing a lot of improvement. She was working with other practitioners to monitor her labs and thyroid medication. She shared that over the last week that she felt like she turned a corner. "I am feeling more like myself this last week. My digestion has greatly improved along with my energy and ability to think more clearly. I am on a small dose of thyroid, which I know is also helping. The 21-Day Program has made such a difference that I plan to stay on it for another twenty-one days. I know that Hashimoto's isn't curable, but with the right tools I can manage it and get it into remission, and that is what I am focusing on right now."

What's Going On

My thyroid threw me into a hormonal hot mess for two years: bone-crushing fatigue, crippling brain fog, wildly erratic periods, terrible constipation, icy hands and feet, and baffling weight gain around my middle. Girl, if this sounds like you, I know exactly how you feel! Or, maybe you're struggling with acne, dry skin, headaches, joint and muscle pain, anxiety, insomnia, or any of the other 300-plus (!) signs that your thyroid has been compromised.

There are this many symptoms because your entire body depends on your thyroid. Every single cell in your body has receptors for thyroid hormone. It is responsible for the most basic aspects of our body's function, impacting all major systems. Thyroid hormone directly acts on the brain, the GI tract, the cardiovascular system, bone metabolism, red blood cell metabolism, gallbladder and liver function, steroid hormone production, glucose metabolism, lipid and cholesterol metabolism, protein metabolism, and body temperature regulation. See what I mean?

The sad fact is that many of us are dealing with thyroid issues whether we know it or not. It's estimated that one in eight women will develop a thyroid condition during her lifetime, with women being five to eight times more likely than men to have one.

The menopause connection. What you need to know is this: The chances of developing a thyroid issue during perimenopause and menopause go up, as this period of transition can be especially rough on this little butterfly-shaped gland at the front of your neck; 26+ percent of women near or in menopause struggle with a thyroid issue. Why? Estrogen dominance significantly reduces the amount of thyroid hormone available to cells, and too much estrogen can block thyroid hormone receptors. In either case, nothing is necessarily wrong with your thyroid gland, but thyroid hormone isn't getting where it's needed and you'll experience the symptoms of hypothyroidism, or an underactive thyroid.

Another reason we're more likely to experience a thyroid issue during this time is because the thyroid is on the front line of lifestyle and environmental threats. It is highly susceptible to poor diet, stress, toxins, and other root causes. Your thyroid gland will take a big hit before a lot of other parts of your body do, and now, during a time when a lot of ignored or suppressed health issues bubble over, it'll be the first to cry out for help.

The autoimmune connection. The most common cause of a thyroid issue is an autoimmune disease, when the immune system targets the thyroid gland and directly impairs its function. The two most common thyroid autoimmune diseases are Hashimoto's and Graves' disease. In Hashimoto's, the immune system attack causes low thyroid function, or hypothyroid. In Graves' disease, the opposite occurs, and the thyroid is overactive, or hyperthyroid.

Inflammation is one of the main drivers of autoimmunity, and we already know that inflammation is a major problem for most of us. It can be fired up by every root cause, including toxins, gut issues, trauma, stress, infections, and nutrient deficiencies. And estrogen dominance yet again plays a role. Excess estrogen is highly inflammatory. The hormonal imbalances you're likely dealing with during perimenopause and menopause, from erratic estrogen to dysregulated cortisol and insulin, contribute to a potential autoimmune attack on your thyroid.

How Do I Confirm It's My Thyroid?

Symptoms of a thyroid condition greatly resemble those characteristically associated with perimenopause and menopause. Doctors hear brain fog, fatigue, and weight gain, and boom, it's "just that time." The very real possibility of a thyroid condition is overlooked or dismissed. Or your doctor may listen to you, but do only what he or she knows to do: check your TSH levels. And that just isn't enough. The range of symptoms and inadequate testing can make diagnosis challenging at any time of life, but it can be more difficult during perimenopause and menopause.

Hormone replacement may be necessary, but the first step should always be to determine why you're experiencing symptoms in the first place. Maybe the reason is estrogen dominance and not an underactive thyroid gland after all. Sometimes addressing the underlying cause of the thyroid problem is enough to resolve it without resorting to thyroid hormone replacement.

If you've been diagnosed with a thyroid condition, you're probably taking steps to correct it and the suggestions in this chapter will support you. The Hormone Makeover Program in Part III will also help to support your thyroid function.

If you haven't been diagnosed but are experiencing symptoms, I encourage you to consider getting a full thyroid panel (See The Importance of Testing on page 284 for the tests you should get) and having the results interpreted by a functional medical practitioner. There is no one perfect way, no one symptom or test result, that will properly indicate how to proceed with treatment for your thyroid issues, whether hyper- or hypothyroidism. The key is to look at the whole picture—your symptoms and your blood tests—and then decide how to proceed. As always, working with a trusted healthcare practitioner experienced in ordering these tests and interpreting the results can provide a more comprehensive picture of how your thyroid is functioning.

Either way, read on to learn more about what might be causing your symptoms—it's more than "the Change"—and how to start addressing them. As you will see, there are a good many things that can impede optimal thyroid function.

Why It's Happening

Yup, your symptoms are linked to your thyroid function and thyroid hormone levels. Not much of an eye-opener there. But you may be shocked by some of the root causes. There are a good many not-so-obvious ways to impede the optimal functioning of this gland, throw your hormones into a tailspin, and leave you vulnerable to thyroid autoimmune conditions, such as Hashimoto's and Graves'.

Too Much Thyroid Hormone

An overactive thyroid, or hyperthyroidism, will produce too much thyroid hormone. Signs of hyperthyroidism include anxiety, insomnia, racing heart, rapid weight loss despite excess hunger, tremors, hot flashes, and high blood pressure. The most common cause is Graves' disease, an autoimmune disease in which your immune system attacks the thyroid and causes it to make more thyroid hormone than your body needs. Over time, the thyroid gland enlarges and swelling behind the eyes may occur, resulting in bulging eyes and vision changes. Thyroiditis, inflammation of the thyroid gland, or an overactive thyroid nodule are other less common causes.

Conventional medicine generally offers only medications, radiation, and surgery to treat the symptoms of an overactive thyroid. Instead, by taking care of the potential underlying root causes, you can often reverse Graves' disease without such harsh measures.

Not Enough Thyroid Hormone

There are two main reasons why your thyroid may be hypothyroid and not producing enough thyroid hormone. One is if you're not getting enough iodine, necessary for the production of thyroid hormones. Iodine isn't produced by the body, so we need to be sure we're getting enough from sources such as seaweed, seafood, dairy, eggs, sea salt, or supplementation to avoid deficiency. The second is if your immune system attacks and damages your thyroid, compromising its ability to produce enough hormone. This is called Hashimoto's, and it's a major cause of hypothyroidism. Seventy-five percent of those with Hashimoto's are women, and that statistic covers only those who have been officially diagnosed.

By diminishing the body's sensitivity to insulin and ability to detoxify estrogen, hypothyroidism contributes to estrogen dominance, a situation many women in perimenopause and menopause are struggling with. This is bad enough on its own, as estrogen dominance brings a host of unpleasant symptoms, but it can also amplify symptoms of hypothyroidism. As mentioned earlier, excess estrogen lowers the amount of available thyroid hormone and blocks receptors. If you're already not producing a lot of thyroid hormone, this scenario limits its supply and impact even more. And excess estrogen boosts inflammation, intensifying the blow to the thyroid from Hashimoto's.

Addressing nutrient deficiencies, lowering inflammation, and getting estrogen dominance under control are just a few ways to address the root causes driving low thyroid function before deciding to use hormone replacement therapy.

Stress

Stress has a direct impact on your thyroid function and does a number on your thyroid hormones. Stress is *not* fuel, no matter what society may lead you to believe. Nope, stress is not going to charge you up for bigger and better success. You know what stress will do? Put the brakes on your thyroid. Put simply: Cortisol is your thyroid's kryptonite. When cortisol goes up, your body shuts down your thyroid gland in order to slow metabolism and conserve fuel for when you might really need it.

Unfortunately, powering down thyroid function doesn't just slow your metabolism, contributing to low fat burn and potential weight gain. Remember how many systems rely on thyroid hormone to function? Every single cell in your body has thyroid hormone receptors, and during states of prolonged stress, your cells can shut thyroid receptors down, lowering cellular metabolism. With a low-functioning thyroid and not enough thyroid hormone to go around, every aspect of your physical and emotional well-being will feel the negative impact.

Cortisol also hikes up inflammation, compromising your immune system and opening the doors for developing an autoimmune thyroid condition. It also promotes insulin resistance by raising blood sugar. Some studies have shown insulin resistance damages thyroid cells and worsens Hashimoto's.

Managing stress is a nonnegotiable when it comes to thyroid health.

Gut Issues

Poor gut health, whether due to leaky gut or an imbalanced gut microbiome, provokes your immune system, accelerates inflammation, and heightens your risk of an autoimmune thyroid condition such as Hashimoto's or Graves'. It's why so many people with thyroid issues also have gut issues.

When it comes to leaky gut, many foods can incite inflammation and make your gut more permeable, such as soy and processed foods, but gluten and dairy are the ones that can do the most damage to your thyroid. The gluten and dairy that make your gut leaky will also increase the likelihood that you'll develop an autoimmune thyroid condition because of how closely the gliadin molecule of gluten and the casein protein in dairy resemble the body's thyroid tissue. As more gluten and dairy leak into your bloodstream, your immune system amps up its attack on the look-alike molecules of your thyroid. These attacks may diminish thyroid function (Hashimoto's) or step it up (Graves' disease). After my Hashimoto's diagnosis, I cut out gluten and dairy as well as other inflammatory foods like unhealthy fats (margarine and vegetable oils, for example), refined carbs, grains, processed meats, and sugary foods to help my body start to heal. After cutting these foods from my diet, I was amazed at how quickly I began to feel like myself again. While some foods can be reintroduced in your diet, gluten and dairy may need to stay out if you have an autoimmune thyroid condition. One bite of gluten can set your body back six to eight weeks in filtering out all of the antibodies it has produced in the battle against your thyroid.

An imbalanced gut microbiome drives inflammation and leaky gut while compromising thyroid function more directly. This means that if your gut isn't in good condition, you are open for a wide variety of issues. Low microbe diversity, or an off-kilter amount of "good" to "bad" bacteria in the gut, reduces thyroid hormone levels by interfering with the conversion of inactive T4 hormone into active T3. With about 20 percent of this conversion happening directly in the gut, anything that throws it off will exacerbate your symptoms. Gut dysbiosis also impairs thyroid hormone receptors, preventing thyroid hormone from accessing cells all over the body for optimal function.

Finally, when the gut is inflamed, cortisol levels rise, and from the section on stress, we know that diminishes thyroid function. An irritated gut can't absorb nutrients as well as it should, leading to thyroid issues once again. Iodine, selenium, iron, and zinc are vital for thyroid health, and while you may be eating enough of these essential vitamins and minerals, your gut can't absorb them properly if it is compromised. And if your body can't get them, then they cannot support thyroid function.

Toxins

The buildup of toxins could be slowing your thyroid down and causing a host of possible hypothyroid symptoms. Studies have found that more than 150 household chemicals can have a direct impact on your thyroid health and hormone balance. Most of these toxins function as endocrine disruptors, mimicking thyroid hormone and blocking hormone receptors, preventing natural hormone from entering the cell. Others damage the thyroid gland directly. Doing some serious targeted detoxification was a major part of my healing journey with Hashimoto's, and I already lived a pretty clean lifestyle! Diving in deeper was a major win in my success story. While autoimmune thyroid disorders can be caused by many different things, up to 20 to 30 percent of them can be linked to toxins. What you put on and in your body on a daily basis greatly impacts your health. A big part of being the CEO of your own healthcare is being the guardian of what enters your body and your home.

Reducing our overall toxic load for hormone balance is integral for healing, so it's time to make over your household. It's not so much about picking and choosing the toxins to avoid as it is about lowering our overall exposure. Pay particular attention to the following, as they have a direct impact on the thyroid:

- Fragrance
- Oxybenzone, in sunscreens
- BPA
- Nonstick surfaces, such as Teflon

- Perchlorate, a chemical used in industry and fertilizers, herbicides, and pesticides
- Heavy metals

Chronic Infections

Your immune system mounts an amazing level of attack when detecting foreign invaders, kicking into high gear to fight infectious agents such as viruses, bacteria, mold, and parasites. The problem is that, while it's running wild to try to defeat the invaders, it can mistakenly start attacking healthy cells and tissues, including those of your thyroid. This threatens your thyroid function and increases your chances of developing an autoimmune thyroid disease. Candida and other forms of yeast overgrowth, small intestinal bacterial overgrowth (SIBO), hepatitis C, and Epstein-Barr virus (EBV) are a few of the infectious agents linked to thyroid issues. Working with your healthcare provider to test for these may help you to identify a hidden trigger for your thyroid issues.

What You Can Do to Support Your Thyroid

It bears repeating: Your perimenopause or menopause symptoms could very well be a thyroid problem, so it's paramount that we make sure this gland is in tip-top condition and do all we can to support it. I know I really struggled before my Hashimoto's diagnosis, feeling like I was going crazy and my body was falling apart. Getting to the root of the problem with nutrition, self-care, stress management, and detox helped me to reclaim control, and it will help you, too. Even if you don't have symptoms, loving your thyroid daily will help to support your body's overall function.

While research on the use of essential oils for thyroid support and healing is ongoing, the evidence strongly supports their ability to alleviate symptoms and support your overall well-being. The following essential oil blends, supplements, herbs, and self-care rituals are specifically designed to promote thyroid health and ease some of the most common symptoms of thyroid imbalance. Use these in concert with the Hormone Makeover Program in Part III and turn to the chapters on stress and digestive issues for more help targeting those root causes.

Top 5 Essential Oils for Thyroid Support

1. Myrrh
2. Frankincense
3. Turmeric
4. Clove
5. Lemongrass

Essential Oil Blends

Diffuser Blends

Overwhelm Busting Diffuser Blend

2 drops Lavender essential oil
2 drops Frankincense essential oil
1 drop Geranium or Roman Chamomile essential oil

Energy Boosting Diffuser Blend

2 drops Bergamot essential oil
2 drops Lemongrass essential oil
2 drops Peppermint essential oil

Rollerball Blends

Thyroid Love Rollerball Blend

5 drops Frankincense essential oil
5 drops Turmeric essential oil
5 drops Myrrh essential oil
4 drops Lavender essential oil
3 drops Lemongrass essential oil
Carrier oil of your choice

Apply 2–3 times each day over your thyroid gland to reduce inflammation and balance your thyroid.

Thyroid Cooling Rollerball Blend

5 drops Peppermint essential oil

5 drops Lemongrass essential oil

5 drops Frankincense essential oil

5 drops Myrrh essential oil

5 drops Clove essential oil

Carrier oil of your choice

Roll over your thyroid on your neck in the morning and at night to support healthy function.

Thyroid-Supporting Supplements and Herbal Remedies

Let me be the first to say that in some cases, thyroid medications are absolutely necessary. I am currently taking thyroid hormone to support optimal thyroid function! There is no shame in including this in your plan to restore thyroid function when recommended by your trusted healthcare provider.

However, for many of us who have milder forms of thyroid dysfunction or are just looking for ways to prevent an issue before it starts, here are some natural supplements and herbal recommendations to set your body up for success. I suggest these in addition to the supplements I recommend for everyone as part of the 21-Day Makeover Plan (page 272).

Supplements

SELENIUM (200 MCG/DAY)

Selenium is a mineral that your thyroid requires to metabolize thyroid hormones. Supplementing with selenium is an important way to prevent the start or progression of thyroid diseases. Whether you have Hashimoto's, Graves', hypo- or hyperthyroidism, selenium supplements can help normalize your thyroid's function and restore your body to balance.

ZINC (30 MG/DAY)

Zinc is involved in multiple levels of thyroid hormone production, regulation, and metabolism, so it is vital to get enough of it to support your overall balance. Foods rich in zinc include some meats, legumes, seeds, nuts, shellfish, and even dark chocolate. However, supplementing is the easiest way to ensure you're getting what you need!

ESSENTIALLY WHOLE® THYROID SUPPORT

Your thyroid is one of the most important endocrine glands, regulating metabolism, energy, and digestive function. Supporting your thyroid with daily nutritional support is a crucial step to restoring your thyroid's health. Essentially Whole® Thyroid Balance is formulated with the perfect balance of essential vitamins, minerals like selenium, chromium, zinc, and manganese to support your thyroid's ability to function optimally and ensure proper conversion of T4 to T3.

MYO-INOSITOL (500 MG/DAY)

Myo-inositol plays an important role in signaling your thyroid to produce its hormones. Supplementing is a great way to support your body, especially if you are facing autoimmune issues or hypothyroidism.

Herbs

ASHWAGANDHA (300–500 MG/DAY)

An adaptogenic herb with powerful cortisol-lowering qualities, ashwagandha can support the health of your thyroid gland. Research has found that taking ashwagandha daily improves TSH, T3, and T4 levels for people with hypothyroid.

Note: Ashwagandha is a member of the nightshade family, so use caution if you are sensitive to nightshades.

HOLY BASIL (1,100–2,900 MG/DAY)

Holy basil—the "Queen of Herbs" in Ayurvedic medicine—supports your thyroid by decreasing stress, lowering cortisol, regulating glucose and insulin, and allowing your body to detox.

Dr. Mariza's Hormone-Loving Rituals and Protocols

Love your thyroid by lowering your stress, address nutrient gaps and regulate insulin levels. Follow the stress-releasing Hormone-Loving Rituals on page 87 and add the necessary supplements and Thyroid Love Rollerball for extra thyroid support.

Chapter 10

Digestive Issues

Rosa, age fifty-six, came to me experiencing daily gas and bloating after lunch and/or dinner. She also reported four to five bowel movements each week and was afraid it wasn't enough given how much she was eating. She shared with me that she felt irritable, stressed, and tired and didn't feel like exercising, even if it helped her digestion and mood. "I feel wiped out all of the time and I think it may be related to what I am eating. I'm tired of my bloated stomach every night before bed; it makes me not want to go to work at the hospital the next day. I've been a nurse for over thirty years, so I should be able to figure this out. I want to feel better, but don't know how to start. I've never had such extreme gut issues as I do right now, and I read all of the time that my gut health is important."

Rosa, who entered menopause five years prior, presented with gut dysbiosis, constipation, and higher than normal levels of stress and exhaustion due to digestive distress.

My recommendations were as follow:

- Eight daily supplements: a multivitamin, 4,000 IU vitamin D, 400–600 mg magnesium citrate (before bed), methylated B vitamins, 250 mg choline with inositol, 2 capsules Essentially Whole® Gut Restore supplement, and 2,000 mg omega-3 fatty acids to increase cellular energy, ease digestive upset, and support healthy blood sugar levels.

- For added gut support: digestive enzymes 15–30 minutes before a meal to aid in digestion and a probiotic (30–50 billion CUFs).
- The 21-Day Hormone Makeover Meal Plan to eliminate inflammatory foods, heal the gut and liver, and support cellular energy.
- Add a morning green smoothie (recipes begin on page 308) with 1–2 scoops of fiber (5–10 g).
- Increased hydration with water with lemon squeezed in the morning and afternoon to improve energy and gut motility.
- Mindfully chewing food to help the digestive process more efficiently.
- To reduce gas and bloating after each meal, use the Happy Gut Rollerball Blend (page 178) before and after eating.

Within ten days, Rosa experienced one bowel movement per day. Her energy levels increased in the afternoon and her bloating was completely gone. She also started walking outside during her lunch break at the hospital. She lost six pounds during the first ten days and it gave her the confidence to keep going. She noticed that most of the weight came off around her midsection. She shared the big needle movers for her so far. "Remember when I told you it was the food I was eating that was causing my bloating; now I know it's true. You made me eliminate so much of my current diet, and I know that it was probably all the dairy or grains. I am incredibly relieved now that I am going to the bathroom every morning. I love that I am moving my body again, I thought I had given that up. And I am pleased with the loss in belly fat. I know belly fat is a precursor for heart disease and diabetes. I'm also enjoying my Happy Gut blend. I have been using it after lunch and dinner just in case. And I am planning to stay on your Makeover Program for another one to two weeks. Why not? My results so far have been great and I want to see how much better they can be."

What's Going On

Too many of us live every single day with all sorts of digestive distress and bathroom worries, including constipation, gas, bloating, heartburn, diarrhea, and stomach pains. We shrug it off as something we ate or a "weak" stomach. Hear me out: Knowing where all of the bathrooms are at your favorite haunts, carrying flushable wipes, planning your day around bowel movements, and being well acquainted with plungers and laxatives is anything but normal.

Sure, the natural hormonal fluctuations associated with your menstrual cycle play a role. Cells lining your entire gastrointestinal tract, from your mouth, down through the esophagus, stomach, small intestine, large intestine, and out the anus, have receptors for both estrogen and progesterone, and they have a huge impact on how it functions, affecting how quickly food moves through the system and how much fluid you retain. It's why you may have experienced regular bouts of bloating, constipation, and loose stools before or during your period. And, it's why in perimenopause and menopause, as these hormone levels became erratic and eventually lower, you may be noticing changes in this pattern, differences in your bowel movements, and more bloating, gas, and constipation.

But shifting estrogen and progesterone don't tell the full story. Any type of hormonal imbalance will have an effect on gut function. If your thyroid is off balance, cortisol is dysregulated due to stress, or insulin is up and down on a sugar roller coaster, your gut health will get axed. And it works both ways, as your gut is directly involved in hormone production, metabolism, and conversion. Gut health is critical to hormone health and vice versa. If left unchecked, poor gut health can lead to a laundry list of chronic health problems: inflammatory bowel disease (IBD), autoimmune diseases such as rheumatoid arthritis and Hashimoto's, diabetes, anxiety, depression, asthma, and eczema.

No wonder, given your gut's starring role in so many essential functions:

Absorbs nutrients. You're not so much what you eat as what your gut can actually absorb. A gallon of green juice and a fistful of supplements won't help you if poor absorption is preventing your body from accessing the nutrients it needs.

Makes and regulates hormones and neurotransmitters that im-

pact gut function, mood, and nearly every aspect of your health. I'm talking about estrogens, thyroid hormones, melatonin, and serotonin, just to name a few.

Affects estrogen levels. Not only does your gut make the three different kinds of estrogen (estrone, estradiol, and estriol), but also a specific group of microbes called the estrobolome that metabolizes excess estrogen, reducing its harmful side effects and helping clear it from the body. An imbalanced estrobolome puts you at risk for estrogen dominance because instead of leaving the body, all of that excess estrogen goes right back into circulation.

Shapes mood. Your gut plays a massive role in emotional well-being. The gut and brain constantly communicate. A troubled gut can send an SOS to the brain that triggers mood changes, anxiety, and sadness, and a stressed, worried brain can initiate pain, "butterflies," or nausea in the gut. Plus, serotonin, the "happy chemical," is one of the most important neurotransmitters for regulating our mood and almost all of it is produced in the gut. If the gut isn't making enough, your brain and mood will suffer. Low serotonin is associated with anxiety and depression.

Supports your immune system. Your gut contains 60 to 80 percent of your immune system, meaning that if your gut is compromised, you'll have a tough time fending off infections and illness. A weakened immune system opens the door to autoimmune disease, including those that attack the thyroid.

Spotlight: Serotonin

Serotonin supports a good mood, but what you may not know is all of the work it does in your gut. It influences gut motility, or how fast food moves through your system. Too much serotonin and things move along too quickly, leading to diarrhea and loose or watery stools. Too little and it's constipation time. Serotonin controls your digestive juices and affects how sensitive to pain, fullness, and nausea you are. Remember the last time you were laid low with food poisoning? It was a flood of serotonin that kept you on the toilet, expelling the contents of your intestines to get rid of the bacteria making you sick. Most serotonin—over 90 percent—is produced in your gut, so a healthy gut equals balanced serotonin, better bowels, and better moods.

Why It's Happening

Quickly offered a prescription by doctors, we often desperately take medications to deal with the symptoms of digestive distress. Anything to end those horrific, embarrassing symptoms, right? But here's the hard truth: Gut issues aren't simple. There is no magic pill to take. They are *not* healed overnight. And most medications simply relieve the symptoms rather than deal with the issue at hand. For lasting health and wellness, it's better to understand the possible hormonal imbalances at play and address the root causes.

Low Estrogen

In perimenopause, estrogen levels may fluctuate wildly, creating symptoms within the body. During periods of low estrogen, the body may respond with constipation, dry stools, bloating, and gas. This may sound all too familiar to those of you in menopause, when estrogen levels reach their more stable low levels.

One of estrogen's many jobs is to keep your stress hormone cortisol levels low. However, as estrogen decreases, cortisol naturally increases. This slows the digestive process (your body always chooses survival over digestion!), extending the time it takes for food to break down and travel through the colon. Gas can build up, causing uncomfortable bloating and flatulence. The more time waste spends in the colon, the more water leaches out and the harder and drier stool becomes, making it more difficult to pass.

Low estrogen also decreases the amount of bile produced by the liver. Bile aids digestion and lubricates our small intestines, so without enough bile to move things along, stool accumulates. This leads to bloating and constipation, a horrible duo that causes pain as it moves through your intestines. And as if that weren't bad enough, less bile also equals more flatulence.

Low Progesterone

Progesterone is a natural muscle relaxant, so when levels are high, your muscles are loose, allowing for easy movement of waste along your pipeline. For this reason, many women struggle with constipation right after ovulation when progesterone levels are low, just beginning their natural rise. In perimenopause and menopause, progesterone levels decline, so you may experience more loose stools, diarrhea, or bloating as bowel activity adjusts.

Thyroid Hormone Imbalance

Thyroid issues are common in women during perimenopause and menopause, with an imbalance in thyroid hormones often the source of digestive problems. Thyroid hormones directly influence metabolism and digestion. Too much (hyperthyroidism) may speed things up, resulting in diarrhea and indigestion, while too little (hypothyroidism) slows things down, causing constipation, stomach pain, and bloating.

Several studies have linked thyroid issues with an increased likelihood of developing digestive issues, including celiac disease and IBD. One of the most interesting discoveries is the connection between hypothyroidism and SIBO, small intestinal bacterial overgrowth, a serious condition that causes pain and diarrhea and significantly compromises the health of the gut microbiome. This study found that more than half (54 percent) of people with a low-functioning thyroid also tested positive for SIBO. We can't overlook the gut when healing the thyroid.

Stress

When you're stressed, do you reach for a candy bar, bowl of ice cream, or other sugary quick-fix snack to boost energy? How about coffee? Alcohol? Energy drinks? Sugar. Sugar. Sugar. Carbs. Carbs. Carbs.

When stress gets high, our bodies switch to binge mode to help ourselves cope and feel better. But why? Because our bodies have increased levels of cortisol telling us we're in danger and food is in short supply. Famine mode! So, what do we do when we see food? EAAAAT! We crave sugar-filled, carb-rich foods to give us a kick of serotonin and boost our low mood.

Problem is, stress has kick-started our fight-or-flight response and stalled our digestive system in favor of dealing with the immediate threat. Our gut is already in crisis dealing with reduced blood flow and motility. The onslaught of serotonin in the gut leaves us with a litany of digestive issues. Over time, our gut lining weakens, increasing gut permeability and leaky gut. Sigh. And the dominos start to fall . . .

Our gut microbiome suffers as well. Stress alters gut bacteria, encouraging the growth of pathogenic bad ones, such as *E. coli,* salmonella, and pseudomonas, which can overrun your microbiome. Gut bacteria take another blow because poor sleep harms them, too, and we all know how hard it is to rest when we're stressed out. In one study, after just two nights of only four hours of sleep, there was an increase in the abundance of bacteria associated with weight gain, obesity, and type 2 diabetes. The body responds quickly!

And the hits just keep on coming. Stomach acid normally prevents you from developing infections and food poisoning by killing harmful bacteria before they make it into the small intestine. But stress can lower its production, making you more susceptible to gut infections. Low stomach acid is also linked to low digestive enzyme production, which helps with the food processing. Secreted by the pancreas into the small intestine to break down proteins, fats, and carbs from foods, digestive enzymes rely on a balance just like the rest of the digestive system. Running low makes it difficult to fully digest your meals and absorb nutrients, promotes the growth of "bad" bacteria, and causes gas, bloating, and indigestion. Hello again, embarrassing symptoms!

The gut is *highly* sensitive to stress—the gut-brain connection is no joke—and getting a handle on it is a priority for good digestion and happy hormones.

Diet High in Processed and Inflammatory Foods

Consuming processed, nutrient-poor food, such as those that contain refined white flour, corn, sugar, and partially hydrogenated oils, alters your gut microbiome, promotes intestinal permeability, and fans the flames of inflammation. Industrial seed oils, the highly processed oils made from soybeans, corn, rapeseed (the source of canola oil), cottonseed, and safflower seeds, are common hidden offenders linked to gut inflammation and the growth of bad bacteria. In addition, artificial sweeteners, food additives, and preservatives are also toxic. The American diet high in refined sugars, carbs, and alcohol feeds those lurking infections deep in your gut as well, nurturing nasties like Candida and SIBO. Yeast and bacteria live on sugar! A lot of harm lurks in the food that we choose to eat.

Eating foods that our body does not tolerate well is another source of inflammation. Certain foods cause an inflammatory response not just in the gut but in the whole body, resulting in painful joints, brain fog, and even headaches and migraines. When you have a food intolerance, symptoms usually begin within a few hours after eating the problem food. Yet, symptoms can be delayed by up to forty-eight hours and last for hours or even days, making the offending food especially difficult to pinpoint. The top food intolerances are: dairy, eggs, corn, soy, gluten, sugar, peanuts, caffeine, and nightshades (eggplant, white potatoes, goji berries, chili peppers, bell peppers, and tomatoes).

One of the best ways to discover if you have a food intolerance is to do the 21-Day Hormone Makeover Program in Part III, using your Food Journal (see page 281) to track your progress. In the program, you will eliminate certain foods from your diet and slowly reintroduce each one back, monitoring your symptoms to determine if it's a problem for you.

Paying attention to what you put in your mouth is the first step toward reclaiming control of your digestive system. Avoiding processed foods and your food intolerances while eating an organic plant-based whole food diet high in fiber and grass-fed animal protein will help keep your gut functioning by supporting a healthy microbiome, preventing leaky gut, and enabling proper nutrient absorption.

Gut Infections

There are loads of different types of bacteria, viruses, and parasites that can wreak havoc on your digestion, creating uncomfortable symptoms including cramps, diarrhea, nausea, and vomiting. A leaky gut with a sickly microbiome is particularly vulnerable to issues.

Candida, an overgrowth of the yeast *Candida albicans,* is one of the most common, as yeast can linger long after you treat it in your reproductive organs. That said, if you frequently find yourself with vaginal yeast infections that never seem to be resolved, chances are you have Candida lurking in your gut. The normal antibiotic treatment can kill the healthy bacteria in your microbiome as well as the bad, so taking probiotics and adding healthy bacteria via fermented foods during treatment can help prevent this cycle from perpetuating.

Another is SIBO, when "healthy" bacteria normally found in the large intestine begin to grow in the small intestine, feeding on carbs and generating excess gas. Think belching, flatulence, and severe bloating.

A few others include the *E. coli* and salmonella bacteria; noroviruses (the most common cause of foodborne illness worldwide) and rotavirus; and the giardia and cryptosporidiosis parasites. These invaders change your gut microbiome for the worse, promote leaky gut, and put your immune system on high alert.

Toxins

Toxins are everywhere, and they exact a high price from our gut. Environmental toxins, such as BPA and phthalates, inflame the gut, increase harmful gut bacteria, and promote leaky gut.

Many of us don't think of antibiotics as a toxin, but they are toxic to your gut microbiome. Doctors are quick to prescribe antibiotics to kill a pesky infection, and let's face it, we're often quick to demand a quick pill fix. But overuse allows bacteria to become resistant to their positive effects and, in many cases, antibiotics aren't needed. Shockingly, according to the CDC, only one in three antibiotics prescriptions are medically necessary, making overprescription a worldwide crisis. Antibiotics fight the bad bugs, but they also kill the healthy bacteria in our guts at the same time, wiping out the balance in our gut. Now our microbiome is weakened, leaving us with embarrassing symptoms and vulnerable to attack by more viruses and bacteria. One quick-fix prescription can do a lot more harm than good. Oh, and don't forget all of the antibiotics we regularly consume from conventionally produced meat, poultry, and dairy that can overwhelm our system. This constant barrage is bad news all around.

What You Can Do to Support Your Gut

It should be crystal clear that we need to do everything we can to promote the healthy functioning of the whole digestive system. Reducing stress, elevating our diet, and avoiding toxins are musts. The following essential oil blends, supplements, herbs, and self-care rituals are specifically designed to restore your gut health. Use these in concert with the Hormone Makeover Program in Part III to lessen symptoms of nausea, relax and soothe irritated bowels, and fight against digestive imbalance. Also turn to the chapters on stress and sleep for more help targeting those root causes.

1. Peppermint
2. Ginger
3. Fennel
4. Cardamom
5. Clove

Essential Oil Blends

Rollerball Blends

Happy Gut Rollerball Blend

6 drops Ginger essential oil
6 drops Fennel essential oil
5 drops Peppermint essential oil
5 drops Clove essential oil
Carrier oil of your choice

Roll over your gut to promote healthy digestive function.

Overindulge Rollerball Blend

10 drops Peppermint essential oil
10 drops Fennel essential oil
Carrier oil of your choice

Roll over your gut to soothe the symptoms of indigestion.

Bloat-Be-Gone Rollerball Blend

10 drops Peppermint essential oil
5 drops Fennel essential oil
5 drops Cardamom essential oil
Carrier oil of your choice

Roll over your belly to ease bloat and gas.

Soothe and Move Rollerball Blend

7 drops Cardamom essential oil

7 drops Ginger essential oil

5 drops Peppermint essential oil

Carrier oil of your choice

Roll over your abdomen to balance your bowel movements.

Gut-Supporting Supplements and Herbal Remedies

As you may expect, the primary way to support your gut's health is through the foods you eat. In the Hormone Makeover Program in Part III, I'll go into much more detail about how you can make choices that lower inflammation, protect your gut, and fuel your health.

Supplements and herbs are a way to quickly bridge the gap to support your digestive health as you begin to heal your body. In addition to the supplements I recommend for everyone in my Foundational Daily Hormone Support Protocol and the Gut Restore Add-On Protocol as part of the 21-Day Makeover Plan (page 272), here are some more recommendations.

Supplements

FIBER (30 G/DAY)

A majority of women in our stage of life are getting *less than half* of the fiber they need each and every day. It helps keep you regular, cleans out the toxins that accumulate in your gut, and plays a crucial role in feeding your microbiome to ensure it stays in a healthy balance. Working a dietary fiber supplement into smoothies is an effortless way to make sure you're getting what you need! Essentially Whole® Pure Daily Fiber is my preferred fiber because it won't cause the bloating and gas that so often accompany fiber powders.

ZINC (30 MG/DAY)

Zinc is an important mineral for many systems in your body, but it is especially critical for maintaining a healthy gut barrier. If you have leaky gut or Crohn's disease, research indicates that zinc is an effective way to strengthen your intestinal walls to ease your symptoms and promote your gut health.

NAC (N-ACETYLCYSTEINE) (1,800 MG/DAY)

NAC is the supplement form of the amino acid cysteine, which is found in high-protein foods. It is a powerful antioxidant that fights against cellular damage and supports immune health. NAC supports your body's detoxification pathways, fighting inflammation and protecting your liver from damage caused by toxins or hormone excess. It also breaks down biofilms in the gut, supports insulin sensitivity, and improves the function of your immune system.

VITAMIN D (4,000–5,000 IU/DAY)

Vitamin D has powerful anti-inflammatory properties to promote your gut's health. People who get higher levels of vitamin D have fewer reports of inflammatory bowel disease, Crohn's disease, and other digestive diseases. It is also necessary to keep your microbiome healthy, which has a major impact on your immune system, hormones, brain health, and more.

Herbs

ALOE VERA (300 MG, TWICE PER DAY)

Packed with essential nutrients, antioxidants, and vitamins A, C, and E, aloe vera provides unparalleled gut support. It soothes and restores balance to your intestines by promoting healthy mucus and bacteria balance that can be depleted by inflammation, leaky gut, and poor diet choices. It also eases constipation by increasing the water content in your intestines. If you suffer from Candida overgrowth or IBS, aloe vera can help control your symptoms naturally.

SLIPPERY ELM (1–3 TSP POWDER 3 TIMES PER DAY, MIXED INTO HERBAL TEA OR WATER)

Another powerful tool to combat inflammation, slippery elm powder supports your gut's health by reducing bloating, relieving digestive discomfort, and easing constipation. If you have IBS or suffer frequent bouts of constipation, slippery elm is an effective treatment to soothe your symptoms and improve digestive regularity.

MARSHMALLOW ROOT (2 G, 3 TIMES PER DAY)

By easing inflammation in your gut, marshmallow root is a powerful remedy to support your digestive healing. Its properties have been found to soothe discomfort, minimize ulcers, and promote regularity by easing both diarrhea and constipation. It works by restoring the function of your gut cells and providing a healthy mucus coating to keep things moving and provide relief, especially if you're dealing with ulcerative colitis or Crohn's disease.

GINGER (2 CAPSULES OF DRIED GINGER [1 G/CAPSULE] TWICE PER DAY)

Ginger is one of the most well-known herbal digestive aids. It has powerful antioxidant and anti-inflammatory properties to treat the root of your gut issues, while its soothing properties combat nausea and overall stomach upset. If you suffer from chronic indigestion, one common root cause is your stomach emptying too slowly. Ginger can speed up the rate at which your stomach empties to alleviate this discomfort.

DANDELION (*TARAXACUM OFFICINALE*)
(DOSAGE DEPENDS ON THE FORM
OF SUPPLEMENT YOU CONSUME)

Though most of us see dandelions in our yard and consider them weeds, they pack a punch for your digestive health. Dandelion root contains a fiber that is a powerful supporter of your microbiome and also helps ease constipation. It also is packed with polyphenols and antioxidants to support the health of your cells and reduce inflammation. Dandelions contain compounds that support insulin sensitivity and promote liver health to enable your body to digest efficiently and put the foods you eat to use to fuel your cells. It's also helpful if you find yourself bloated throughout your cycle by reducing the fluid buildup in your body.

There are many ways to consume dandelion: capsules, tablets, tinctures, teas, and even dandelion root coffee.

Note: Dandelion is a member of the ragweed family, so if you are allergic, proceed with caution.

Dr. Mariza's Hormone-Loving Rituals and Protocols

Digestive Massage Ritual

Any of the rollerball blends in this chapter can be used for gentle digestive massage, around the belly button, though I recommend starting with Peppermint. Or experiment to find the individual oils and blends that complement your needs the best. You don't have to wait until things get bad to try a digestive massage while lying down in bed in the morning or at night. Know that digestion can be supported from your esophagus down through the trachea to the large intestine. Massage the oils into your skin around your belly button with smooth, circular motions, and when you're finished add a warm, wet compress to push the oils in deeper.

Castor Oil Pack for the Gut

Castor oil packs are a powerful way to provide sustained digestive health support. The ricinoleic acid in castor oil can soothe the bowel, while its undecylenic acid fights internal fungal issues and other potential infections. Pelvic pain and cramping of any kind can be eased by the healing support of castor oil, especially when combined with essential oil support, as the oils can both be absorbed transdermally. Use castor oil packs two to three times a week for up to ninety minutes each, with a rest day in between. (Note: Castor oil packs can increase menstrual flow.) Check out the Resources section for where to buy my favorite one.

Sip Digestive Teas

Herbalists have been recommending tinctures and teas for digestive unrest and soothing for centuries, so if you haven't tasted these delicious alternatives to water, it is time to do so! Digestive tea supports your body's hydration and keeps your stool soft. Rich in antioxidants, polyphenols, and other herbal constituents, teas nourish the body while also supporting your healthy gut flora.

Drinking these teas at a certain time each day will help your mind and body to come to expect this step in your digestive routine. I recommend trying several to find the one that works the best for you. My favorites are ginger, green, chamomile, peppermint, dandelion (avoid if you have a ragweed allergy), fennel, tulsi (holy basil), and Pu'er tea.

Chapter 11

Brain Fog
and Cognitive Function

Candace was forty-eight when she came to me concerned with recent trouble focusing and recalling full sentences during presentations at work. A project manager for a Fortune 500 company, she felt like she was losing her edge. She had always been the go-to person to manage multiple projects without skipping a beat, until recently. "It's like the words vanish into thin air. It has never happened to me before, and now I find it happening once a week at least. I need to get my brain back on track. My sleep is okay, but isn't great, and I work pretty late hours most days of the week. With juggling my family and work obligations, something has to give, and it's usually sleep. I am taking some supplements, but I am drinking coffee to get me through most of the day. Is it all catching up to me? How can I change my schedule and my priorities?"

Candace presented with brain fog, low progesterone levels due to perimenopause, and decreased cortisol levels in the morning and afternoon.

My recommendations were as follows:

- Six daily supplements: a multivitamin, 2 capsules Essentially Whole® Adrenal Love supplement, 400 mg magnesium glycinate, 15 mg zinc, 500 mg rhodiola, 2,000 mg omega-3 fatty acids to lower stress levels and support brain function.

- The 21-Day Makeover Plan to remove any foods that could cause brain fog, inflammation, and support healthy hormone changes.
- Add green smoothie to breakfast or lunch with 6–9 grams of maca.
- Increase water intake by carrying a 22-oz water bottle and re-filling 2–3 times at work.
- Substitute green tea for coffee and cut out snacking in the afternoon. The L-theanine in green tea reduces stress without causing sedation.
- For afternoon slumps, incorporate Instant Brain Power Roller-blend (page 195) every hour or diffuse energizing essential oils such as Peppermint and Grapefruit.
- A 20-minute Nighttime Ritual, including a sleep meditation before bed to relax the mind before sleep.
- Start each morning with a 5-minute meditation and Wake Up Energized Rollerball Blend (page 133) to help with stress and provide mental clarity at the start of the day.

Within about a month, Candace found herself back in the game. Her work recall improved significantly. She had changed her schedule to make room for a morning and evening ritual, and it made a massive difference. She lost eight pounds by Day 19 on my program and experienced more energy, especially after taking three-minute mini-breaks throughout her workday with the Wake Up Energized Rollerball Blend. I asked how she felt overall. "I didn't know that brain fog was caused by inflammation. I have a feeling all the coffee, bars, and quick meals contributed to my inability to focus. Having a cleaner diet has helped me out tremendously. I am also sleeping better and setting myself up to get better quality sleep. Lastly, the oils make a huge difference throughout the day. Why didn't I know about these before? That little extra break in my day with the oils jolts me up in a good way. I always use my Wake Up Energized blend before a meeting or presentation, and I feel much more focused and clear."

What's Going On

You charge into a room, but forget what you were doing. You zone out during meetings or important conversations. Certain words elude you, even though you know they are right there on the tip of your tongue. You recognize the person's face but cannot recall her name. Memory issues, trouble focusing, a lower attention span, and an overall sense that your thinking just isn't as sharp all fall under the umbrella term of "brain fog." Many women come to me complaining of this fogginess during perimenopause and menopause, most of them in a hot panic that it means they are slipping into dementia, or one of its most common types, Alzheimer's disease. Rest assured, very rarely is this the case, even in situations where there's a family history.

A certain amount of memory issues are age-related. As your body ages, so do the blood vessels and brain cells, or neurons, that your brain relies on to transmit information. They don't communicate as well with each other, causing brain function to slow down—a bit. It may take you a little longer to recall information, learn something new, or screen out distractions, but there's no reason to expect significant memory or cognitive decline as we age if we take care to keep our bodies and brains healthy. This is a use-it-or-lose-it situation and lifestyle factors significantly influence our ability to think clearly.

And so do our hormones, especially estrogen and progesterone, which is why about 60 percent of middle-aged women report difficulties with concentration and brain function. This number spikes during perimenopause due to the erratic fluctuations of estrogen and decline of progesterone. Recalling words, relying on verbal memory, becomes increasingly difficult as hormone levels decline into menopause. And the other symptoms associated with these hormonal changes, such as hot flashes, night sweats, and insomnia, lead to poor sleep and fatigue, two issues known to cause fuzzy thinking no matter what your age. Mood issues such as anxiety and depression, a higher risk for women during this time of change, can also make it tough to focus, process new information, and feel mentally sharp.

Here's the good news: Brain fog can be addressed naturally, and it doesn't need to be a lasting issue. One study found that women struggled most with brain fog during the first year of menopause, but their symptoms improved over time. Living a lifestyle that consistently supports hormone balance while keeping your mind active will help to clear the fog.

SIGNS OF BRAIN FOG	SIGNS OF DEMENTIA
Occasionally forget where you left your keys or glasses but find them later.	Regularly lose items and never find them.
Occasionally forget an appointment or walk into a room and forget why you entered.	Forget how to do things you've done many times, such as pay bills or get dressed.
Able to remember and describe incidents of forgetfulness.	Can't recall or describe specific instances where memory loss caused problems.
Become easily distracted or have trouble finding the right word or name during a conversation.	Unable to hold a normal conversation. Words are frequently forgotten, misused, or garbled, and phrases and stories are repeated in the same conversation.
Judgment and decision-making ability is the same as always.	Routine lack of judgment and poor decision-making; behave in socially inappropriate ways.

Unlike the brain fog associated with perimenopause and menopause, dementia and Alzheimer's get worse over time. See your doctor right away if you recognize some of the signs of dementia in yourself or a loved one.

Why It's Happening

Your brain relies on the right balance of hormones to function optimally, and I don't just mean estrogen and progesterone. If cortisol, insulin, and thyroid hormone, among others, are skewed, you'll struggle to be clearheaded. Since daily habits play a huge role in our cognitive function, there are a number of possible root causes for brain fog. A few top offenders are detailed below, but anything that causes inflammation in the body is a threat. Chronic inflammation doesn't just wreak havoc on your hormones, it can create gaps in the blood–brain barrier, allowing toxins to slip through and inflammation to spread through your brain. What do you get when that happens? Brain fog.

Low Estrogen

Estrogen is critical for learning and memory; your brain is *packed* with estrogen receptors. Many are found in the hippocampus and prefrontal cortex, parts of the brain associated with short-term memory, verbal memory (recalling words), planning, and decision-making. When these receptors don't get their fill due to the ups and downs of estrogen production during perimenopause and the lower estrogen levels of menopause, you have the telltale symptoms—memory lapses, trouble making choices, difficulty putting pieces of information together and recalling that word on the tip of your tongue. Estrogen also helps direct blood flow to the parts of the brain that need it, but a lack of proper blood curbs cognitive function.

Women who have had their ovaries removed before menopause nearly double their risk of developing cognitive issues, with the chances increasing as the age of removal lowers. The sudden decrease in estrogen is thought to be a major reason. If you are facing hysterectomy, I recommend discussing with your trusted healthcare provider the benefits and risks of your ovaries also being removed.

Low Progesterone

Recently, scientists have realized just how critical progesterone is to brain health and clear thinking, reasoning, and remembering. It influences the growth, development, and repair of brain cells. It can also protect the brain from damage, reducing swelling after injury and myelination, the process of forming a protective sheath around a nerve to maintain a seamless flow of communication between neurons. Because perimenopause and menopause bring a natural decline in progesterone, some brain fog is to be expected. An overabundance is a sign of a larger issue.

Too Much Cortisol/HPA Axis Dysfunction

We often hear the expression that "stress kills," and in the case of your brain cells, it's literally true. A burst of cortisol in a fight-or-flight moment may sharpen your thinking and enhance your ability to consolidate short-term memory, because you need total focus when your survival is at stake. The problem lies in chronically elevated cortisol levels, which damage the structure of the brain and rewire its communication network, creating lag time and difficulty in accessing, contextualizing, storing, and retrieving long-term memories. In short? Brain cells die off, aging the brain prematurely.

It doesn't help matters that cortisol also lowers the rate at which new brain cells are generated. Over time, if cells become resistant to cortisol and HPA axis dysfunction is in full swing, cortisol isn't able to enter cells and work its anti-inflammatory magic. Increased brain inflammation increases the symptoms of brain fog. And you are left searching vainly for the right word or feeling forgetful.

Thyroid Hormone Imbalance

Brain fog and cognitive difficulties are symptoms of both an underactive and an overactive thyroid. Memory problems, especially related to verbal memory, difficulty concentrating, and small changes in executive functioning (planning, impulse control, and decision-making) are linked to hypothyroidism. People with hyperthyroidism may have trouble concentrating, slower reaction times, and decreased spatial organization skills.

Brain fog was one of the first symptoms I experienced before I was diagnosed with low thyroid function. On multiple occasions, I would be in an interview and out of nowhere would forget what I was going to say, as if the words just disappeared into the air. Luckily, once I got my thyroid issue under control, these symptoms improved, and yours will, too, if you suspect a thyroid imbalance.

Dysregulated Insulin and Blood Sugar

Running primarily on glucose, your brain is your most energy-demanding organ, using up nearly 50 percent of all of the sugar in the body. Thinking, learning, and memory all rely on a sufficient supply. Not enough and the brain slows, resulting in poor attention and forgetfulness, an all-too-familiar feeling that hits around three p.m. I know it well, when I hankered for that granola bar and diet soda to get me through the rest of the day. For years, I let this pattern control my afternoons, relying on sugar and caffeine to give me that extra boost. The brain is tricky, leading us to believe we need sugar to spike our levels back up. The truth is that our brains can maintain until dinner if we fuel it with the right foods at breakfast and lunch. When we cave to those sugar cravings, we do more harm than good.

Too much sugar inflames the brain, contributing to irritability, mood swings, and brain fog. Over time, chronically high blood sugar levels lead to insulin resistance within the body. Insulin strengthens the synaptic connections between brain cells, helping them to communicate better and supporting the development of strong memories. When insulin levels in the brain decrease due to insulin resistance, cognition can be impaired. Research has linked both a diet high in sugar and insulin resistance with an increased risk of developing Alzheimer's and other forms of dementia.

Chronic blood sugar imbalances can also mess with neurotransmitters such as serotonin that help keep our moods stable, opening the door to depression and anxiety, and making it even tougher to plan, remember, and pay attention.

Stress

Stress makes it harder to think, reason, and focus. In survival mode, your brain is laser-focused on the perceived threat and not interested in learning new information or thinking too deeply. As we've seen, stress can cause a fluctuation in several hormones, including cortisol and insulin, that have a direct impact on cognitive function. Stress can also cause your hippocampus to shrink, limiting your short-term memory, and fans the flames of inflammation in many ways. Not only does it slow down the liver's detoxification process, allowing more toxins to make their way into the bloodstream, but it can also cause "leaky brain," when the blood–brain barrier, the protective layer, allows toxins to pass through and cause damage. And stress is just plain exhausting! When you're physically and mentally spent, brain fog sets in big-time. Additionally, chronic stress can damage mitochondrial function, eventually causing exhaustion, fatigue, mood swings, and fogginess. Without high-functioning mitochondria, we lack mental resilience.

Poor Sleep

A lack of quality sleep will make your thinking cloudy, and fatigue and exhaustion are two of the biggest offenders when it comes to confusion and inattention. Sleep deprivation disrupts our brain cells' ability to transmit information, leading to feelings of fogginess. It also causes a variety of hormonal imbalances that lead to brain fog, like ramping up cortisol and suppressing the production of the neurotransmitter dopamine. This crushes your mood and destroys your motivation. We're at greater risk for sleep apnea in menopause as well, and it's crucial to get it treated immediately.

Gut Issues

Gut inflammation, whether due to leaky gut or an imbalanced gut microbiome, equals brain inflammation. So interdependent is the gut–brain relationship that research even shows leaky gut can *cause* leaky brain, or permeability of the protective blood-brain barrier, leading to even more inflammation and damage. Avoiding inflammatory foods, such as processed foods and food intolerances (gluten and dairy for many people), will help to lift brain fog. When you eat a food you are sensitive to, the immune system releases inflammatory compounds called cytokines to manage the situation. But cytokines also attack brain tissue, with high levels found in those with Alzheimer's disease. In addition, poor gut health means your brain is not getting all of the nutrients it needs for optimal functionality. A deficiency in iron, vitamin B12, omega-3s, or vitamin D, among others, contributes to brain fog, something I experienced firsthand. Support your gut, your second brain, and you support focus, attention, and all-around mental clarity.

Toxins

We are exposed to so many toxins, contaminants, microbes, and chemicals each and every day that it is no wonder we all have a high toxic load. And while regulations say a minute exposure to one particular toxin is not detrimental to human health, we have to consider the multitudes of exposures over many years, which almost definitely can have adverse influences on our natural physiological processes. This usually stems from an inflammatory response to these exposures. Our immune systems can withstand and tolerate quite a few assaults, but sometimes we are simply not strong enough to handle the overstimulation of our immune systems. This leads to chronic inflammation of our critical organs, including our gut and brain. An inflamed brain can't function at its best, kick-starting a domino effect in the body.

What You Can Do to Support Brain Health and Cognitive Function

Luckily, we can move the needle on brain fog symptoms. For mental clarity, I highly suggest employing essential oils for immediate results. Simply inhaling or diffusing these oils can enhance your alertness and concentration, as well as rid the body of brain fog and mental chatter. The following essential oil blends, supplements, herbs, and self-care rituals are specifically designed to decrease inflammation in the body and support the immune system to help clear cloudy thinking. Use these in concert with the Hormone Makeover Program in Part III to boost attention, memory, and learning. Also turn to the chapters on stress, sleep, and digestive issues for more help targeting those root causes.

Top 5 Essential Oils to Enhance Cognitive Function

1. Rosemary
2. Peppermint
3. Basil
4. Frankincense
5. Vetiver

Essential Oil Blends

Diffuser Blends

Instant Focus Diffuser Blend

2 drops Frankincense essential oil
2 drops Peppermint essential oil
2 drops Rosemary essential oil

Memory Boost Diffuser Blend

2 drops Rosemary essential oil

2 drops Wild Orange essential oil

2 drops Frankincense essential oil

Personal Inhaler Blends

Mental Alert Inhaler Blend

6 drops Grapefruit essential oil

3 drops Basil essential oil

3 drops Rosemary essential oil

2 drops Frankincense essential oil

Afternoon Recharge Inhaler Blend

6 drops Frankincense essential oil

6 drops Lavender essential oil

6 drops Vetiver essential oil

Aromatic Sprays

Focus and Uplift Room Spritz

3 drops Bergamot essential oil

3 drops Rosemary essential oil

3 drops Peppermint essential oil

3 drops Vetiver essential oil

Distilled water or witch hazel

Spritz in the air or on your clothes for sustained focus and an energy uplift.

Rollerball Blends

Laser Focus Rollerball Blend

5 drops Basil essential oil

5 drops Peppermint essential oil

5 drops Rosemary essential oil

5 drops Grapefruit or Wild Orange (optional)

Carrier oil of choice

Apply to temples and massage gently twice a day.

Instant Brain Power Rollerball Blend

10 drops Tangerine essential oil

5 drops Spearmint essential oil

5 drops Frankincense essential oil

3 drops Cedarwood essential oil

Carrier oil of choice

Roll on pulse points as needed throughout the day.

I've Got This Rollerball Blend

8 drops Wild Orange essential oil

5 drops Peppermint essential oil

4 drops Clary Sage essential oil

2 drops Sandalwood essential oil

Carrier oil of choice

Roll behind ears, on back of neck, and on wrists and inhale as needed.

Brain-Supporting Supplements and Herbal Remedies

Treating the root causes to clear brain fog is the best way to support mental clarity and optimal brain function. But there are many brain-boosting supplements and herbs to help raise your game while improving mitochondrial health and immune function. In addition to the supplements I recommend as part of the 21-Day Makeover Plan (page 272), here are some of my favorites.

Supplements

ESSENTIALLY WHOLE® NEURO+ SUPPORT

Neuro+ Support is a supplement that combines many powerhouse ingredients to energize your brain and improve your memory and ability to think, while addressing some of the root causes behind your brain fog. These include acetyl-L-carnitine to give your cells their energy, repair damaged brain cells, and improve your ability to learn and remember; and citicoline to supply materials to your brain cells that they use to communicate with one another.

VITAMIN D (4,000–5,000 IU/DAY)

Your body creates vitamin D when you expose your skin to direct sunlight; however, around 40 percent of people are still deficient in vitamin D. Vitamin D is one of your body's first lines of defense. Having enough vitamin D is essential for optimal bone and arterial health. This power-packed hormone protects your brain cells from developing plaque and damage that can lead to dementia and Alzheimer's. To ensure optimal absorption, choose a vitamin D3 supplement with vitamin K.

PHOSPHATIDYLSERINE (100 MG, 3 TIMES/DAY FOR A TOTAL OF 300 MG/DAY)

Your brain cells rely on phosphatidylserine to communicate. Supplementing with it promotes your ability to focus and remember while protecting you from degeneration that can result as you age. It also limits and controls the release of cortisol to help your body rebalance from its stressed-out state.

Herbs

RHODIOLA (START AT 50 MG/DAY AND STEADILY INCREASE UNTIL YOU ACHIEVE DESIRED RESULTS, BUT DO NOT EXCEED 680 MG/DAY)

Rhodiola is an adaptogenic herb that helps to increase serotonin levels, which can improve your overall mood and may improve your reasoning skills as well. It can enhance energy metabolism and increase the capacity of your mitochondria to produce energy-rich compounds in the brain, as well as in the rest of your body. It can also protect you against physical and mental stress, fatigue, toxins, and more.

BACOPA MONNIERI (300 MG/DAY)

This adaptogenic herbal supplement has been used for thousands of years in Ayurvedic practices because of its brain-boosting power. It can help balance your dopamine and serotonin levels, can promote memory, and may even alleviate some depressive tendencies. It also can cut down on the inflammation that causes your brain to become foggy and confused and which can accelerate cognitive decline.

Just know that this is not an immediate, quick-fix solution. Consistently using it for four to six weeks and incorporating it into your lifestyle is the way you'll get the most out of this powerful herb!

MATCHA

Formulated from the whole leaf, matcha delivers 100 percent of the nutrients and benefits of green tea. Packed with powerful antioxidants and other health-promoting compounds, matcha helps rid the body of free radicals that attack your cells. These free radicals can cause significant damage to brain cells, which impairs your ability to think, reason, and remember. Matcha also provides the body with L-theanine, which is an amino acid that boosts mental clarity—even if you just have one cup per day.

CURCUMIN (200–500 MG, TWICE/DAY)

Found in turmeric, curcumin increases blood flow to the brain to promote clear thinking and maintain the health of your brain cells. Unlike other supplements, curcumin provides almost immediate memory-boosting benefits. A study found that Alzheimer's patients experienced a boost in memory and retention in as little as an hour after taking curcumin, in addition to improved mood and stress levels. Be sure to your choose a supplement free of artificial fillers or additives.

RESVERATROL (150–450 MG/DAY)

Resveratrol is a powerful anti-inflammatory and antioxidant compound that supports your brain's health. Although it is found naturally in red wine, grapes, and some other foods, resveratrol supplements pack a much bigger punch for your health. Research indicates that it can ward off signs of aging, including cognitive decline. It also prevents damage to your brain cells and inhibits the formation of plaques that are the hallmark of Alzheimer's.

GINKGO BILOBA (40–120 MG, 3 TIMES/DAY)

Ginkgo has been used for more than 5,000 years in Chinese medicine. By increasing circulation to your brain, ginkgo biloba supplements maintain the health of your brain cells to boost your memory, prevent declines related to dementia and Alzheimer's, and even balance neurotransmitter and hormone levels that exacerbate your symptoms.

PANAX GINSENG (400 MG/DAY)

The anti-inflammatory properties of *Panax ginseng* reduce feelings of fatigue and stress and boost cognitive function, focus, and memory.

Dr. Mariza's Hormone-Loving Rituals and Protocols

Reducing stress boosts memory, focus, and concentration. Follow the stress-releasing Hormone-Loving Rituals and Protocols on page 87, especially meditation and prayer to refocus your mind. Use the Instant Focus or Memory Boost diffuser blends for extra support. In addition, try the following.

Musical Support Ritual

Music is my secret strength for supporting cognitive function and focus, as the brain needs the left hemisphere for lyrical focus while the right side loves a good melody. Music speaks to my soul, and I love having a good playlist for impromptu stress-busting dance parties. But how do I use it to strengthen my brain? Memorizing song lyrics and busting them out whenever I need a boost. Singing makes my heart *and* my brain happy.

Challenge yourself with a new playlist of songs that you don't know by heart. Throw in a few fast-paced lyrics to really get your mind pumping, and dare yourself to learn it by a certain time. One of my latest obsessions is learning all of the lyrics in the Tony Award–winning musical *Hamilton*. Use the music you love to light your brain up.

Chapter 12

Low Libido and Vaginal Dryness

When she was about fifty-seven, Lydia read *The Essential Oil Hormone Solution* and got in touch with me to see if I had any specific recommendations for her vaginal dryness and low libido. She had already been diagnosed with vaginal atrophy and had been given a natural estradiol cream (Estrace), but she was interested in what else she could do to support her sex life with her partner. "I rarely engage in sex anymore because it's so painful and irritating. The pain immediately turns me off and I want to just read a book, or watch a movie. No surprise that it's having an impact on my relationship. We've been together a very long time, so he's understanding, but I can see he's frustrated and I feel so bad about that. Besides the local estrogen, I don't know what to do. I need to know that this isn't the end for me. I also don't want to be on estrogen forever at my age, even if it's applied topically."

Lydia presented with a classic case of low estrogen due to being in menopause for more than five years.

My recommendations were as follow:

- Five daily supplements: a multivitamin, 200 IU vitamin E, 2 capsules Essentially Whole® Hormone Balance supplement, 400 mg magnesium glycinate, and 2,000 mg omega-3 fatty acids to support hormones, energy, vaginal health, and cellular longevity.

- Drink ginseng tea, or take 3–5 grams red ginseng daily.
- Add a green smoothie to breakfast or lunch with 6–9 grams of maca.
- Use a natural lubricant with essential oils (page 211) for less friction during sex.
- Apply the Sexual Energy Rollerball Blend (page 209) to boost libido and sensual emotions.
- Self-care rituals: unlimited intimacy by hugging, kissing, and bedtime conversation, a Nighttime Ritual with a relaxing bath and diffusing essential oils to help get in the mood for intimacy. Set the mood with music, diffuse the Deep Connection Diffuser Blend (page 208), and participate in a couples massage.

Within six weeks, Lydia wrote back to me with good news: "The estrogen cream is definitely working for me. I have noticed a boost in my libido overall. I think the magnesium, vitamin E, and Hormone Balance are helping with other menopausal symptoms, too, including low energy and hot flashes. All of a sudden my hot flashes and night sweats have stopped after I started taking the supplements. I'll take my wins any way I can get them. I have really enjoyed the natural lubricant over a store-bought brand. The biggest shift for me is with the rituals. I felt so closed off, but now I am making a big effort to spend time and create intimate moments and I am really enjoying them. It doesn't always lead to sex and I am okay with that. I love the connection and conversations. The oils smell amazing and they add an extra element that I really enjoy. I plan on continuing to use them and the supplements. I am hoping to come off of the estrogen cream soon."

What's Going On

Let me speak some truth: The end of reproductive function does *not* mean the end of sexy time. As you go through perimenopause and menopause, you probably will notice changes in your libido, or your natural sex drive. Some women experience an increase in libido and report that their libido and sex life is the best it's ever been, while other women will experience a decrease in sex drive that impacts their relationships and emotional well-being. They may find they don't become aroused as easily and feel pleasure as intensely; and they experience pain with penetration. But a decline in libido and sexual pleasure is *not* inevitable or necessarily permanent. You do not have to "give up" or throw in the towel on sexy time if you don't want to, for any reason. You can support your body and your libido to have the sex life you deserve.

You should know there are many, many reasons why you may be experiencing low libido. We're quick to blame hormones, especially during the menopause transition, but hormones are only a small part of the full picture that is your sexual health. The fact is, women can experience low libido at any time throughout their life, not just during perimenopause and menopause. In fact, more young women are complaining of low sexual desire. According to one study, one in ten women aged eighteen to forty-four do. So, don't go thinking you're alone in your feelings.

The natural decline in estrogen and testosterone you're experiencing isn't necessarily the reason you're not in the mood. What's probably going on is this: Hormone changes are causing physical changes, like vaginal dryness, that make sex less pleasurable and perhaps even painful. Forty percent of postmenopausal women report pain with intercourse, and of course uncomfortable, hurtful sex will dampen your desire. The good news is that there are several natural options, lubricants, and moisturizers to help ease these physical symptoms and make sex more enjoyable. Just doing that can help boost desire, enabling you to focus more on your partner and less on discomfort.

Maybe you've become so frustrated, you think your sexual health just doesn't matter anymore. Or, it's a lost cause because your prime has passed. Or low libido and vaginal dryness are just how things are for you now. Sometimes it's easier to ignore the problem or say no than try to work with your partner to have a satisfying sex life.

But you should know this: Vaginal health is important no matter what. You should always feel good down there whether you are sexually active or not. And sex is good for you, with or without a partner. Orgasms are good for you, with or without a partner. Expressions of intimacy and intimate touch, whether sexual or not, lower stress, improve mood, preserve heart health, reduce blood pressure, and boost immunity. And if you are in a relationship, sex and intimate touch can deepen your connection with your partner.

Now, in this time of transition, be empowered to revisit your attitudes about sex and focus on what satisfies you, not just what's "good enough." If you're struggling with low libido and/or vaginal dryness, rest assured that you are in good company, and there are things you can do to get yourself back in the mood.

First, let's take a closer look at what's happening with these two frequent complaints.

Low Libido

Are you ready to spice things up, but having trouble feeling connected to your partner or getting yourself to want to have sex? These are signs of a low libido, a common problem for so many women. Other signs are:

- Little to no interest in sexual activity, including masturbation
- Recurring lack of desire
- Lack of interest in your partner's overtures for sexual activity
- Few sexual thoughts or fantasies
- Concern about your lack of sexual desire and interest

So many women are in this boat. Despite what our seemingly sex-crazed society often leads us to believe, most women are not in sexual overdrive. Between the demands of life, career, and often motherhood, we find ourselves lacking the spark, the energy, or the drive to fulfill our intimate needs. The sad reality is that sex frequently gets pushed to the bottom of our to-do lists; and let's face it, how often do we actually get to complete everything on our list by the end of the day? And yet I hear it all the time: It's not just a matter of having enough time for a roll in the hay, it's about having the desire to do it.

This is especially the case during perimenopause and menopause. Growing priorities and hormone changes lead to fatigue, overwhelm, and low libido. Very often, it seems like finding your libido will take more effort and energy than you have to give. Then there are the other factors that play a role: the values you were brought up with, the quality and connection in your relationship, how much stress you are dealing with each day, how much deep, restful sleep you are getting, and how you are feeling emotionally. It may also take more time and foreplay for you to reach orgasm, and, once you get there, your orgasms may not be as intense. Your clitoris may seem less sensitive than it used to be. Your vagina may feel dry, itchy, and less elastic, making sex uncomfortable or painful. You may be having more frequent urinary tract infections (UTIs). Or you may be dealing with pelvic pain. All of this (and more) will influence your libido.

Vaginal Dryness

It's hard to be interested in sex if it's uncomfortable or painful, am I right? Many women around menopause experience vaginal dryness, and it is the ultimate libido crusher, squashing desire, arousal, and satisfaction. But this isn't just about sex. Vaginal dryness with its itching, burning, irritation, even bleeding, doesn't feel good at any time and can negatively impact your overall quality of life and emotional well-being.

So, what's going on? It's actually a simple answer: Your vagina is changing. As estrogen levels fall during late perimenopause and menopause, the tissue in your vagina becomes thinner and less able to lubricate itself, making it more susceptible to inflammation and irritation. And you're not alone in this. At least half of us will experience some degree of vaginal dryness; in fact, one study found that 75 percent of midlife and menopausal women reported that vaginal discomfort negatively affected their sex life.

That said, the natural shift in estrogen levels is not the only reason you may be experiencing vaginal dryness or painful sex. You'll want to work with a trusted healthcare provider to rule out other possibilities such as an injury or trauma, skin condition, infection, allergic reaction, sexually transmitted disease, pelvic floor dysfunction, endometriosis, and uterine fibroids.

Why It's Happening

Declining hormones can cause physical symptoms that create vaginal dryness and contribute to low libido. But there are a lot of other factors at work that we have more control over. Stress, lack of sleep, poor diet, and lack of exercise not to mention the quality of our relationship, our level of self-confidence, and body image can have a tremendous impact on our libido, and we can absolutely do something about those!

Decreasing Levels of Estrogen, Testosterone, and DHEA

The vulva and vagina rely on estrogen, so declining levels can make the vaginal walls thinner, less elastic and lubricated, and more inflamed. The healthy bacteria in the vagina also rely on estrogen, and an imbalance in the vaginal microbiome can lead to dryness, burning, and irritation.

Testosterone is involved as well, as levels decrease naturally over time; we have about half as much in our fifties and sixties as we did in our twenties. Estrogen is made from testosterone, so when testosterone declines, estrogen levels decline, too. Testosterone triggers the hypothalamus to prepare your erogenous zones for sexual activity, which is why achieving orgasm may take longer now. It's thought that testosterone plays a role in female sex drive, but it's unclear just how much of one or exactly how it works. Several studies have found no difference in testosterone levels in women who have high levels of desire and those diagnosed with a desire disorder. So low testosterone does not necessarily mean low libido.

DHEA is needed to make both estrogen and testosterone, so not enough of this precursor hormone can compromise the body's ability to produce the other two.

Thyroid Hormone Imbalance

Thyroid hormones impact nearly every cell, organ, and system in the body, so it should come as no surprise that an imbalance will disrupt your sexual health. Both hypothyroidism (a low-functioning thyroid) and hyperthyroidism (an overactive thyroid) are associated with low libido and painful intercourse. Other common symptoms of thyroid dysfunction, such as fatigue, can also dampen desire.

Stress and Trauma

Stress is the ultimate libido crusher. In survival mode, your body does not want you getting pregnant—and there goes your sex drive. If you're stressed (or having hot flashes!), you're probably not sleeping well, and fatigue is another serious buzzkill.

If you have experienced trauma or think you have, I encourage you to seek a trained therapist or counselor to help you resolve it for your overall health and well-being, because it may be at the root of your low libido. Any type of trauma, not just sexual, may inhibit sexual desire.

Lifestyle

Poor sleep, a nutrient-deficient, high-sugar diet, lack of exercise, and not enough self-care will affect your sex drive. It's really not about how old you are; it's about how healthy you are. A good foundation of healthy lifestyle practices sets you up for lasting hormone and sexual health and lowers your risk for many chronic conditions. And those chronic conditions, such as obesity, high blood pressure, diabetes, heart disease, and chronic pain, tend to lower libido. Many medications used to treat these conditions do a number on your libido, too. Antihypertensive medications, sedatives, ulcer medications, antihistamines, and antidepressants are all associated with some level of sexual dysfunction. Supporting your pelvic health is important as well, since no one feels sexy worrying about a leaky or overactive bladder.

Other Root Causes

I recommend looking more closely at the other physical, emotional, and social root causes that are contributing to low sex drive. After all, only by identifying them can you work on addressing them. Other contributors include:

- past relationships
- not feeling sexy
- partners struggling with their own sex drive
- emotional struggles, depression, anxiety
- emotional needs not being met
- cultural and social attitudes and religious beliefs about sex
- antidepressants

. . . and the list goes on. Dealing with these issues, admitting them to yourself (journaling helps!), and communicating them to your partner and/or a trusted healthcare provider are essential for getting in the mood.

What You Can Do to Support Libido

You *can* reclaim your sexy by incorporating some simple lifestyle changes with the aid of supplements, self-care, and aromatherapy. Essential oils and sensuality go hand in hand, and they can help get you in the mood and address known libido crushers such as stress and fatigue. Have fun selecting scents that arouse both you and your partner, experimenting with different combinations in preparation for intimacy or during foreplay. Use these blends, supplements, and herbs in concert with the Hormone Makeover Program in Part III to bring more passion and enjoyment back into this area of your life. Also turn to the chapters on stress, sleep, hot flashes and night sweats, and pelvic floor dysfunction for more help targeting those root causes.

If you've tried the natural approach and still need more assistance, check out the additional options for libido at the end of this chapter.

Top 5 Essential Oils to Support Libido

1. Clary Sage
2. Rose
3. Sandalwood
4. Jasmine
5. Neroli

Essential Oil Blends

Diffuser Blends

Deep Connection Diffuser Blend

2 drops Lavender essential oil
2 drops Jasmine essential oil
2 drops Clary Sage essential oil

Sensual Mood Diffuser Blend

2 drops Jasmine essential oil
2 drops Sandalwood essential oil
I drop Ylang Ylang essential oil

Sexy Night Diffuser Blend

2 drops Sandalwood essential oil

2 drops Rose essential oil

2 drops Neroli essential oil

Aromatic Spray

Sensual Awakening Spritz

6 drops Sandalwood essential oil

4 drops Ylang Ylang essential oil

2 drops Jasmine or Rose essential oil

Distilled water or witch hazel

Spritz bedclothes, pillows, and the air to promote intimacy and sensuality.

Rollerball Blends

Sexual Energy Rollerball Blend

15 drops Clary Sage essential oil

10 drops Ylang Ylang essential oil

5 drops Neroli, Jasmine, or Rose essential oil

Carrier oil of your choice

Roll over pulse points and heart to awaken your sexual energy and boost your sensuality prior to intimacy.

Enhanced Sensation Rollerball Blend

3 drops Peppermint essential oil

3 drops Jasmine essential oil

3 drops Ylang Ylang essential oil

3 drops Clary Sage essential oil

Carrier oil of your choice

Roll over pulse points, especially ankles and behind your ears to awaken sexual energy.

Massage Blends

Self-Love Personal Massage Blend

3 drops Ylang Ylang essential oil

2 drops Jasmine essential oil

1 drop Rose essential oil

2 teaspoons of jojoba, sweet almond, or fractionated coconut oil

Inner Thigh High Massage Blend

2 drops Clary Sage essential oil

2 drops Neroli essential oil

2 drops Ylang Ylang essential oil

2 teaspoons of jojoba, sweet almond, or fractionated coconut oil

Mutual Spice-It-Up Massage Blend

2 drops Sandalwood essential oil

2 drops Neroli essential oil

1 drop Cassia or Cinnamon essential oil

2 teaspoons of jojoba, sweet almond, or fractionated coconut oil

Sensual Soak Bath Blends

Couples Time Bath Soak

1 drop Sandalwood essential oil

1 drop Rose or Jasmine essential oil

1 drop Neroli essential oil

1 drop Ylang Ylang essential oil

2 cups Epsom salts

Soak for no more than 20 minutes and enjoy the intimate quiet time together, being sure to pat dry and hydrate well afterward.

Personal Sensuality Bath Soak

2 drops Clary Sage essential oil

1 drop Ylang Ylang essential oil

1 drop Rose or Jasmine essential oil

2 cups Epsom salts

Soak for no more than 20 minutes, allowing your body to unwind and personally prepare for intimacy. Be sure to pat dry and hydrate well afterward.

Natural Lubricant with Essential Oils

$1/2$ cup fractionated coconut oil (liquid coconut oil or MCT oil)

$1/4$ cup aloe vera

1 teaspoon vitamin E oil

3–5 drops essential oils (Frankincense, Lavender, Roman
    Chamomile, Clary Sage, Rose)

In an 8-ounce glass jar, add fractionated coconut oil, aloe vera, and vitamin E. Mix ingredients together well. Add 3–5 drops of essential oil. I personally love to combine gentle floral oils like Lavender and Rose essential oils. Apply before sexual intercourse.

Libido-Supporting Supplements and Herbal Remedies

Since so many of our sexy-time struggles are based around hormone fluctuations, resetting those is going to be your best bet to restore your passion. In addition to the supplements I recommend as part of the 21-Day Makeover Plan (page 272), consider adding the following to help rebalance your hormones and promote sexual health.

Supplements

TOPICAL DHEA

Topical DHEA can counteract the symptoms of age-related skin issues that make sex painful by boosting sebum production to restore a healthy skin texture and relieve dryness.

One of my favorites is Julva by renowned OB-GYN Dr. Anna Cabeca. Known as "The Dream Cream" for good reason, Julva naturally and safely fights aging to rejuvenate, refresh, and repair your lady parts to restore passion and intimacy. It combines DHEA with other natural herbal ingredients to offer you benefits that kick in quickly and last as a long-term solution.

ESSENTIALLY WHOLE® HORMONE BALANCE

Hormone Balance is my own formulation of stellar hormone-loving ingredients in one convenient package, including ingredients such as black cohosh to support vaginal lubrication and elasticity.

Herbs

TRIBULUS (*TRIBULUS TERRESTRIS*) (7.5 MG/DAY)

A natural herbal remedy, Tribulus is a recognized aphrodisiac to improve your sexual experiences. Women who take Tribulus consistently report enhanced desire, arousal, lubrication, and satisfaction with decreased pain.

MACA (1,500–3,000 MG/DAY)

Maca supports healthy hormone balance and reduces your feelings of stress and anxiety in order to make you feel more energized. With stress, fatigue, and hormone dysfunction all impacting your suffering libido, this is an easy, natural addition to your daily routine.

RED GINSENG (200 MG/DAY)

Red ginseng can relax your pelvic and vaginal muscles to help increase your ability to feel arousal and pleasure. Research indicates that oral red ginseng increases libido and sexual satisfaction in menopausal women, without adverse side effects.

Dr. Mariza's Hormone-Loving Rituals and Protocols

Intimate Couples Massage

Touch can make us feel loved and safe. An intimate massage can bring you and your partner close when sex isn't appealing, but it can also be great foreplay to get you primed and in the mood. The key is the release of oxytocin—our feel-good hormone—that comes from the simplest touch to cuddling to hugs to any form of embrace. Since your skin is your largest organ, it makes sense that our sense of touch plays such a large role in intimacy and comfort.

I recommend using a carrier oil such as sweet almond, jojoba, or fractionated coconut oil, and then adding a single essential oil that is mutually appreciated, especially one with aphrodisiacal properties.

Self-Love Ritual

Communication is paramount in every relationship, including the one you have with your inner self. When we feel bad about our bodies, we may find it very difficult to be connected to our partner, especially during moments of intimacy. Your body image is tied to your self-love. Repeating positive affirmations daily can strengthen your foundational self-love just as much as supplements or essential oils. Try repeating, "I accept and love my body unconditionally," during deep breathing exercises and as you look yourself in the eye in the mirror each morning and night. It may feel strange at first, but trust me. The more you repeat it aloud and the more you hear yourself saying it, the more you will eventually believe it. I love coupling this with my favorite Superwoman Rollerball Blend (see page 117) first thing in the morning as I set an intention for my day.

Additional Treatment Options for Libido

If you find that you need more support, consider these options, including several over-the-counter vaginal moisturizers and lubricants available to help make sex more pleasurable.

Vaginal Moisturizers

Try a vaginal moisturizer (K-Y Liquibeads, Replens, Sliquid, others) to restore some moisture to your vaginal area. You may have to apply the moisturizer every few days. The effects of a moisturizer generally last a bit longer than those of a lubricant.

Water-Based Lubricants

These lubricants (Astroglide, K-Y Jelly, Sliquid, others) are applied just before sexual activity and can reduce discomfort during intercourse. Choose products that don't contain glycerin or warming properties, because women who are sensitive to these substances may experience irritation. Avoid petroleum jelly or other petroleum-based products for lubrication if you're also using condoms, because petroleum can break down latex condoms on contact.

Topical Bioidentical Estrogen (Estriol)

This is *not* used to increase systemic estrogen levels, but is used to vascularize (increase blood flow) to the vulva, as well as to thicken it. Vaginal estrogen has the advantage of being effective at lower doses and limiting your overall exposure to estrogen because an insignificant amount reaches your bloodstream.

You insert this cream directly into your vagina with an applicator, usually at bedtime. Typically women use it daily for one to three weeks and then one to three times a week thereafter, but your doctor will let you know how much cream to use and how often to insert it.

Chapter 13

Pelvic Floor Dysfunction, Urinary Incontinence, and Urinary Tract Infections

Patricia found me through a mutual friend and fellow practitioner. When we got on the phone, Patricia explained that for several months she had the urge to pee often during the day. "I can't seem to hold it anymore. I am afraid I am going to pee my pants in public or at work. I feel too young for this. What can I do to address my urge incontinence before it gets worse and I start leaking?"

At age fifty-five, Patricia's issues were clear: urge incontinence, mild anxiety, and pelvic floor dysfunction.

My recommendations were as follows:

- Six daily supplements: a multivitamin, 2,000 mg omega-3 fatty acids, 400 mg curcumin, 4 capsules Essentially Whole® Hormone Balance, 400 mg magnesium glycinate, 1–2 chewable tablets Essentially Whole® Calm & Restore to support mood, hormone levels, and decrease inflammation.
- The 21-Day Hormone Makeover Meal Plan to support a healthy gut and reduce inflammation.
- Refer to a physical therapist or Isa Herrera's Pelvic Pain Relief Program (pelvicpainrelief.com).

- Gradually start Kegels under supervision or guidance to release pelvic discomfort and strengthen the pelvic floor muscles.
- Apply the Pelvic Soothe Relaxation Rollerball Blend (page 223) before going to bed with a gentle pelvic massage.
- Avoid drinking beverages 30 minutes to one hour before bed to reduce getting up at night.

Two months after working through Isa Herrera's program and consulting with her physical therapist, Patricia emailed me with her progress: "Dr. Mariza, my urges are almost entirely gone. I feel less inflamed and I am rocking the Kegels. Overall improvements are improved digestion, little to no urges, and I am experiencing far less panic moments. I feel like I have my body and life back. I will be continuing with many of your recipes, my gut-loving foods, and my physical therapist. I love the Calm and Restore supplement for a quick way to relax my mind and reduce any anxious feelings."

What's Going On

I hear from so many women who plan their days around the availability of a bathroom or wear pads every day to prevent leakage and "just in case." They're worried about having an accident and embarrassed that they have to go so much or unexpectedly. No woman should stop going out or doing the activities she loves—including having sex—for fear of urinary incontinence. I want you to know it's not a natural part of aging or inevitable because of perimenopause or menopause. Urinary incontinence and other bladder-related issues, such as urinary tract infections (UTIs), are often connected to problems associated with the pelvic floor, including weak pelvic floor muscles. The good news is, we have a lot of control over how strong those muscles are.

Pelvic floor disorders are very common. According to a National Institutes of Health study, more than a quarter of women (27 percent) ages forty to fifty-nine are affected by a pelvic floor disorder, with that percentage increasing to 37 percent in women ages sixty to seventy-nine, and to 50 percent in women aged eighty and older. The message to take away from these numbers is not that pelvic floor issues are normal or simply a part of aging, but that far too many of us aren't getting the help we need or accessing the variety of effective treatments available to us. Don't suffer in silence. There's nothing to be embarrassed about here, and you have so much to gain by addressing the situation head on rather than ignoring or "managing" it with an adult diaper. We can significantly improve or even reverse your symptoms and help you get your life back.

Let's take a closer look at what's going on with three of the most common bladder-related issues you may be dealing with: pelvic floor dysfunction, urinary incontinence, and UTIs.

Pelvic Floor Dysfunction

Your pelvic floor muscles create a "sling" or "hammock" extending from your pubic bones at the front of your pelvis to your tailbones at the back. This hammock supports the organs in your pelvis, including the bladder, urethra, uterus, vagina, large bowel, and rectum. By contracting and relaxing these muscles, you control urination, bowel movements, and sexual intercourse, and you want them to be strong and flexible. Pelvic floor dysfunction occurs when these muscles have weakened and you no longer have the ability to control them.

Signs of pelvic floor dysfunction include:

- Frequent urination
- Painful urination
- Leaking urine or stool
- Difficulty evacuating your bowels, constipation, and straining
- Ongoing pain in your lower back, pelvic region, vagina, or rectum
- Painful intercourse
- Pelvic organ prolapse, when one of the organs in your pelvis, such as your bladder, has moved down into the vagina. This can feel like dragging or pressure in your vagina or you may see a bulge at the entrance to or just outside of your vagina.

Why might these muscles lose their tone? Childbirth can stretch and damage the pelvic floor muscles, and if you had an episiotomy, a C-section, or a hysterectomy, you have a higher chance of developing pelvic floor dysfunction. Declining estrogen is also a factor, but there are a lot of reasons related to habit and lifestyle:

- Weight gain or obesity
- A diet high in processed foods, sugars, and carbs
- Not enough exercise
- Smoking and repetitive coughing
- Constipation
- Poor posture (misaligned spine and pelvis)
- Chronic stress

Urinary Incontinence

If you've ever felt like you were going to the bathroom constantly, worried you wouldn't make it in time, or have leaked urine when you laughed or in the middle of yoga class, you know the misery of incontinence. And then there's sex. It's estimated that 1 in 4 women with incontinence avoid intercourse or worry about leakage so much that they can't relax and enjoy sex. Time to get a handle on this!

There are a few different types of urinary incontinence and it's important to know which one you're dealing with:

Stress incontinence. This is the most common type of incontinence, in which urine leaks during activities that stress your musculature, such as coughing, sneezing, laughing, lifting, and exercising. It can be caused by weak pelvic floor muscles and being overweight. Extra weight increases pressure on your bladder and surrounding muscles, weakening them and permitting urine to escape. Vaginal childbirth can also weaken the muscles needed for bladder control and promote pelvic organ prolapse, associated with incontinence. The bladder and uterus are supported by many of the same muscles and ligaments, so any surgery that involves the reproductive system, such as hysterectomy, may damage the supporting pelvic floor muscles and lead to incontinence.

Urge Incontinence. This is when all of a sudden you feel the need to empty your bladder and then, due to an involuntary muscle contraction, a flood of urine is released before you have a chance to get to a toilet. It is most often caused by nerve damage due to diabetes, stroke, a spinal cord injury, multiple sclerosis, Parkinson's disease, or another condition impacting your nervous system.

Overactive bladder syndrome. If you have the urge to run to the bathroom more than six to eight times daily (and no more than once during the night), you may have an overactive bladder. Weak pelvic muscles, nerve damage, excess weight, and a UTI or other infection can all contribute to an overactive bladder.

Urinary Tract Infections

You know the signs: burning and pain during overly frequent urination, itching down there, and cloudy, smelly urine. At one point or another, you've probably had a urinary tract infection (UTI), when pathogens, usually bacteria, infects the bladder, kidneys, or other part of the urinary system. Bladder infections are the most common. About half of all women will have a UTI over the course of their lifetime, and the frequency tends to go up during perimenopause and menopause, with the risk increasing four or five years after your final period. This is due to physical changes, including weak pelvic floor muscles, pelvic organ prolapse, urinary incontinence, thinning vaginal tissue, and trouble completely emptying the bladder. Lower estrogen levels play a role in these physical changes, but strengthening those pelvic floor muscles can go a long way toward reducing the likelihood of a UTI.

Why It's Happening

Bladder issues often have multiple causes, but during perimenopause and menopause we can't overlook the role of declining estrogen and weak pelvic muscles. These are two drivers of pelvic floor dysfunction, urinary incontinence, and UTIs.

Low Estrogen

Estrogen helps keep the muscles and ligaments of your pelvic floor strong, flexible, and resilient. As estrogen levels fluctuate during perimenopause and eventually reach their menopausal low, they become less supple and supportive. This means we have to actively work these muscles to keep them functioning at their max and reduce the chance of developing a prolapse, urinary incontinence, or UTIs.

Estrogen supports a healthy urethra, the short tube that carries urine from your bladder out of the body, and bladder, which is loaded with estrogen receptors. Declining estrogen can impair the seal between your bladder and urethra, resulting in leakage, and thin the lining of the urethra, exacerbating incontinence.

Low estrogen increases your risk for UTIs due to an imbalance of bacteria in the vagina. Estrogen aids the "good" bacteria, helping them to thrive and produce acid, lowering the pH level of the vagina and killing off the "bad" bacteria. With insufficient estrogen, the pH of the vagina rises, becoming less acidic and allowing the "bad" bacteria to proliferate and cause UTIs.

Weak Pelvic Floor Muscles

If strengthening your pelvic floor muscles is not part of your regular exercise routine already, it should be. These muscles regulate urine flow, and if they are weak, you'll likely experience incontinence. The inability to hold urine increases your likelihood of UTIs. Exercises to train and bolster your pelvic muscles, such as Kegels, can support pelvic organs, help maintain bladder support, and help control urinary incontinence. They can also improve the symptoms of pelvic organ prolapse. And stronger pelvic floor muscles may even improve sex, by increasing blood flow to the vagina—good for arousal and lubrication—and sensation through better control of your muscles.

What You Can Do to Support Your Pelvic and Urinary Health

There are many effective strategies to strengthen your pelvic floor, cure or significantly improve incontinence, and cut back on UTIs. The following essential oil blends, supplements, herbs, and self-care rituals are specifically designed to support you. Use these in concert with the Makeover Program in Part III to address the food, diet, stress, and other lifestyle issues contributing to pelvic floor dysfunction. Turn to the chapter on stress for more ways to address that root cause and the one on low libido and vaginal dryness for help targeting that sister issue.

The lifestyle recommendations below and in the Hormone Makeover Program are designed to effectively support your pelvic health, reduce inflammation, and restore your vitality. With that said, I want to encourage you to meet with your trusted healthcare professional and do a full pelvic examination to rule out any other conditions that may be contributing to your discomfort and symptoms.

This is especially important if you are experiencing recurrent UTIs. Make sure that your urethra is evaluated for any evidence of thinning along the outer urethra. If thinning is noticed, consider a topical estrogen to strengthen and thicken the urethra.

How to Support Your Pelvic Floor and Urinary Health with Essential Oils

Essential oils can help support your pelvic and urinary health overall. I recommend using some of the remedies below for sustained support if this is an issue for you, while others are only for temporary usage for more immediate needs.

Try the oils individually to find what works for you, and to discover if you prefer warmth or cooling sensations to relieve pelvic discomfort, or a combination of both. Applying essential oils, massaging them in, and then finishing with a warm or cool compress seems to be the ticket for many women, while others prefer super warm followed by cold.

Top 5 Essential Oils for Pelvic
Floor and Urinary Health

1. Clary Sage
2. Cypress
3. Juniper Berry
4. Lavender
5. Marjoram

Essential Oil Blends

Pelvic Soothe Relaxation Rollerball Blend

7 drops Lavender essential oil
7 drops Frankincense essential oil
7 drops Clary Sage essential oil
Carrier oil of your choice

Massage into the abdomen.

Bladder Support Rollerball Blend

10 drops Cypress essential oil
10 drops Juniper Berry essential oil
Carrier oil of your choice

Roll over bladder 2–3 times a day while problems persist.

Pelvic Pain Massage Blend

2 drops Lavender essential oil
1 drop Clary Sage essential oil
1 drop Marjoram essential oil
1 teaspoon carrier oil

Gently smooth over your abdomen and follow with a hot or cool compress, or both.

Inner Thigh Muscle Massage Blend

2 drops Peppermint or Wintergreen essential oil

2 drops Copaiba essential oil

2 drops Lavender essential oil

1 teaspoon carrier oil of choice

Rub up and down your inner thighs. Use as needed while pain persists.

Pelvic Support Bath Soak

2 drops Lavender essential oil

1 drop Eucalyptus essential oil

1 drop Peppermint essential oil

1 drop Rosemary essential oil

2 cups Epsom salts

Soak for no more than 20 minutes while allowing your body to relax and breathe. Be sure to hydrate well after your soak!

Supplements and Herbal Remedies to Support Pelvic and Urinary Health

In addition to the supplements I recommend for everyone in my Foundational Daily Hormone Support Protocol as part of the 21-Day Makeover Plan (page 272), consider adding the following.

Supplements

VITAMIN D (4,000–5,000 IU/DAY)

Up to 80 percent of us are deficient in vitamin D, thanks to being inside most of the time and wearing sunscreen whenever we do venture out. Research indicates a strong link between vitamin D levels in the body and pelvic health, as well as with overall skeletal and muscular function. When vitamin D levels decrease, there is a much higher chance of developing pelvic dysfunction, prolapse, or incontinence.

Hormone Balance is my own formulation of stellar hormone-loving ingredients in one convenient package. It contains powerful ingredients like black cohosh, chaste tree, DIM, calcium, magnesium, B-complex vitamins, and more to promote hormone balance, healthy muscles, and your overall well-being.

Herbs

There are several herbs with powerful antioxidant and anti-inflammatory properties that can help ease your pelvic pain by cutting down the inflammation that is elevating your symptoms. They include:

Curcumin: 200–500 mg, twice/day

Calendula: Steep 5–10 ml of the herb in 1 cup of boiling water

Quercetin: 1,000–2,200 mg/day

Roman Chamomile: Steep 3 teaspoons in 1 cup boiling water

Each of these is a safe, effective measure you can employ to cut the inflammation that is leading to your pelvic dysfunction, pain, and urinary incontinence.

Dr. Mariza's Hormone-Loving Rituals and Protocols

Daily Kegels

Kegel (pronounced "KAY-gull") exercises, a series of pelvic floor exercises to strengthen and sustain healthy bladder and bowel function, can be done anytime, anywhere, and without anyone else realizing what you are doing. My favorite place to Kegel is in the car at a stoplight! It is important to discuss Kegels with your trusted healthcare provider, as they aren't recommended for everyone, such as women whose overly tight pelvic muscles are causing their issues. For how to do Kegels correctly, check out pelvic pain relief expert Isa Herrera at her website.

Castor Oil Pack

Derived from the castor oil plant *Ricinus communis,* castor oil has been used for centuries to promote healing, specifically in the reproductive and digestive systems. Castor oil itself is widely known for its ability to break up stagnation, inflammation, and toxins. Castor oil packs can help with overall circulation, pain caused by endometriosis, and softening scar tissues from C-sections, surgery, cysts, adhesions, and dysplasia. It also promotes ovarian, uterine, and fallopian tube health by stimulating the lymphatic and circulatory system and removing waste and toxins from the pelvic area.

I recommend using a castor oil pack when you are experiencing pelvic pain and discomfort, amping up the power of your pack by adding essential oils. Check out the Resources section for where to buy my favorite one.

How to Prevent and Relieve Urinary Tract Infections with Essential Oils

While the key to preventing horrible UTIs is proper urinary hygiene (wiping front to back once), sometimes you find yourself dealing with the horrible pain and burning due to a bacterial infection. The most common culprits are *Escherichia coli* (*E. coli*) and *Klebsiella pneumoniae*, though other bacteria and yeasts such as *Candida albicans* and *Candida famata* can be playing a negative role as well.

While many essential oils have been found to play a promising role in eradicating these specific bacteria, the top five that I recommend are my favorites to boost and support both your immune system and your urinary tract and bladder. While Oregano and Melaleuca are great for temporary issues, Clove supports your body year-round. In addition, Grapefruit is a perfect addition to your water infusions. And finally Juniper Berry is excellent for supporting your urinary health in times of need or for an everyday extra boost to kidney function. Try them individually or go for my tested rollerball remedies to find one that works for you and your needs!

Top 5 Essential Oils For UTI Support

1. Clove
2. Grapefruit
3. Juniper Berry
4. Oregano
5. Melaleuca

Essential Oil Blends

Urinary Issues Rollerball Blend

6 drops Oregano essential oil
6 drops Clove essential oil
6 drops Frankincense essential oil
6 drops Lavender essential oil
Carrier oil of your choice

Roll over bladder 2–3 times a day while problems persist. Use for only 2–3 days.

Urinary Health Rollerball Blend

10 drops Juniper Berry essential oil
10 drops Grapefruit essential oil
Carrier oil of your choice

Roll over bladder 2–3 times a day to support your bladder and urinary tract health.

Urinary Soothing Massage Blend

2 drops Melaleuca essential oil
2 drops Lavender essential oil
1 drop Clove essential oil
1 drop Oregano essential oil
1 teaspoon carrier oil of your choice

Carefully massage into your lower abdomen over your bladder or above your kidneys on your back and inner thighs. Lie back and relax your muscles, breathing deeply and allowing the warmth to soothe. Be careful to wash hands well afterward, as Oregano and Clove are both warming oils.

Urinary Soothing Bath Soak

3 drops Melaleuca essential oil
3 drops Juniper Berry essential oil
2 cups Epsom salts

Lie back, allowing your legs to open, and gently clean your urethral opening. Soak no more than 20 minutes, being sure to hydrate well after.

UTI-Supporting Supplements and Herbs

In addition to the supplements I recommend as part of the 21-Day Makeover Plan (page 272), try some of these natural products to treat a UTI head-on and prevent its return instead of jumping straight to antibiotics.

Cranberry extract capsules (or unsweetened cranberry juice). Cranberries contain compounds that prevent bacteria from attaching to your bladder and urethra. If UTIs are a common problem for you, taking cranberry capsules daily can help prevent them from occurring in the first place. They are highly anti-inflammatory, so cranberry is an easy, natural way to relieve your discomfort quickly.

D-mannose (1,000 mg/day). D-mannose is a way to both prevent and treat UTIs. A natural type of sugar found in cranberries, apples, oranges, green beans, broccoli, and more, d-mannose has been found to be as effective as antibiotics at preventing UTIs in women who suffer them frequently. It also can alleviate symptoms to bring you relief faster.

Vitamin C (1,000 mg). Vitamin C, a powerful antioxidant, can create an environment in which the harmful bacteria cannot survive, enabling your body to get rid of them more efficiently.

Uva-ursi tea. A safe and well-recognized UTI remedy, uva-ursi tea can help prevent and treat your symptoms. It calms inflammation and eliminates harmful bacteria that cause UTIs in the first place.

Dr. Mariza's Hormone-Loving Rituals and Protocols

Good Hygiene Protocols

Research indicates that proper urinary hygiene can reduce the incidence of UTIs and other issues. Make sure to follow these best practices for keeping your urinary tract healthy:

- Hydrate frequently in order to void your bladder regularly, every three to four hours.
- Don't hold urine. Go when you feel the urge.
- Wipe once front to back after evacuation.
- Clean genitals daily and after sex, wiping the vulva with a warm washcloth from front to back.

Chapter 14

Heavy Bleeding and Fibroids

When my mom, Jody, was about forty-nine, she started experiencing heavy bleeding accompanied by erratic periods. She was deep into perimenopause and experiencing estrogen dominance, which caused her periods to become very heavy. It got so bad at one point that she used twenty-five tampons to try to address the nonstop bleeding, which led to an emergency visit from a plumber when the tampons clogged her pipes!

Upon closer consultation, my mom had estrogen dominance, perimenopausal symptoms, low cortisol levels in the morning and afternoon, and low progesterone.

My recommendations were as follows:

- Eight daily supplements: a multivitamin, 4,000 IU vitamin D, 400 mg magnesium glycinate, 200 mg chasteberry, 50 mg iron, 100 mg DIM (diindolymethane), methylated B vitamins, and 2,000 mg omega-3 fatty acids to metabolize estrogen, balance her reproductive hormones, reduce stress. and increase cellular energy.
- The 21-Day Hormone Makeover Meal Plan to support liver and gut detoxification pathways and support healthy hormone changes.

- Add green smoothie to breakfast or lunch with 6–9 grams of maca.
- For afternoon slumps incorporate Instant Motivation Roller-ball Blend (page 132) or Wake Up Energized Rollerball Blend (page 133) every hour with one minute of breath work.
- A 20-minute self-care Morning Ritual consisting of inhaling the Instant Motivation Rollerball Blend (page 132) and grati-tude journaling.
- Apply the Slow the Flow Rollerball Blend (page 243) over the lower abdomen during period flows.
- Tennis or 30-minute nature hikes 4–5 times per week.
- A 20-minute Nighttime Ritual, including a 5-minute sleep meditation before bed to relax the mind before sleep.

Four weeks later, after completing the first twenty-one days of the Makeover Program, my mom called me to let me know that her period bleeding was heavy, but not as heavy as the last month. She didn't have a double-digit tampon day and that was a big win for her. She experienced other big wins that she couldn't wait to share with me. "Mariza, guess what? My PMS is definitely better this month. I don't feel like killing anyone. I lost ten pounds and I am continuing the pro-gram for sixty days total because it's not interfering with my tennis. I am sleeping better with the meditation app you told me about and I am taking bath soaks a couple days a week and they are easing my stress. I am loving the green smoothies. They are so easy; you know I love easy food options. And I am loving my oils. The Peppermint has been a lifesaver for my crazy chocolate cravings. Thanks, honey!"

What's Going On

Heavy bleeding, or menorrhagia, is the kind of surprise no one wants, which is why it frustrates me that no one ever tells women that dur-ing perimenopause they will likely experience it. In most cases, this is absolutely normal. In fact, at the very end of perimenopause, there may be so much heavy bleeding that it has a name: flooding. Heavy bleeding and erratic periods occur naturally during this transitional time due to the natural fluctuation of estrogen and progesterone. However, they can be exacerbated by not-so-good lifestyle choices that promote hormone imbalance, particularly estrogen dominance. In addition, uterine fibroids, noncancerous growths of smooth connective tissue and muscle, often appear for the first time in perimenopause or get angry during this time—and are one of the most common causes of heavy bleeding.

There's a lot of misunderstanding out there on these issues that I'd like to clear up so that you can understand what can happen and what falls within the abnormal range.

Heavy Bleeding in Perimenopause

During perimenopause, about 25 percent of women have heavy bleeding, and most women bleed profusely toward the end of perimenopause. Repeated heavy bleeding can lead to iron-deficiency anemia, a lack of iron resulting in not enough red blood cells to carry adequate oxygen to your cells, making you feel tired, fatigued, weak, and dizzy.

Here's what you should keep in mind:

What we mean by "heavy bleeding." Usually, menstrual bleeding lasts about four to five days, with the amount of blood loss being small, about two to three tablespoons. Heavy bleeding is generally considered to be bleeding for more than seven days with twice as much blood loss. Most of us don't measure our blood flow, so if you have to change your "regular flow" pad, tampon, or period underwear nearly every hour for several hours and have to change it during sleep, you're likely in heavy bleeding territory. That said, these are very general guidelines. Only you know what's normal—and abnormal—for you.

For now, an abnormal bleeding pattern may be your new normal. I know this can be unsettling and frustrating. The good news: It will all be over when you stop ovulating and reach menopause! For now, check in with yourself and assess if what you are experiencing is normal for your body. Although new and different bleeding patterns are common during perimenopause, some unusual bleeding can be a sign of a problem that needs medical attention.

Fluctuating estrogen and progesterone is not the only reason you may be experiencing heavy bleeding. Here are some possible other causes.

Fibroids: These are benign (noncancerous) tumors ranging in size from a pea to as large as a basketball and growing anywhere inside or on the uterus. They can grow quickly, especially during perimenopause due to estrogen dominance, the imbalance of estrogen and progesterone. (See "Spotlight: Fibroids" on page 234 for more.)

Pregnancy-related complications: Pregnancy during perimenopause is possible, even if your cycle is irregular. Ectopic pregnancy, miscarriage, placenta previa, and other problem pregnancies can cause irregular bleeding.

Hormonal contraceptives: Birth control pills, IUDs, and other forms of hormonal birth control may cause various irregular bleeding patterns.

Endometrial (or uterine) polyps: These are small, soft benign growths of the uterine lining.

Adenomyosis: The endometrial glands that line the uterus grow into it, causing blood to form in the uterine wall with no easy place to drain, resulting in heavy, painful periods.

Infection: Infections, including sexually transmitted diseases such as chlamydia and gonorrhea, can occur in the vagina, cervix, uterus, fallopian tubes, or ovaries.

Precancerous or cancerous growths: Rare gynecological cancers, such as uterine and endometrial cancer, cause heavy vaginal bleeding.

In most cases, heavy bleeding is an unavoidable part of the transition. I know it sucks, but we can reduce its severity and negative impact on our lives by resolving the estrogen dominance driving it and supporting a healthy foundational lifestyle.

Spotlight: Fibroids

Fibroids, also called leiomyomas, are benign lumps or growths in the uterus. They are very common, and their likelihood increases with age until menopause. Nearly 70 to 80 percent of women are affected by uterine fibroids in their reproductive years. In one U.S. study, Caucasian women showed an incidence of uterine fibroids of 40 percent by age thirty-five and almost 70 percent by age fifty, while Black women had an incidence of 60 percent by age 35 and over 80 percent by age fifty. You may not even know you have them. They cause symptoms, such as heavy bleeding, about 20 percent of the time. Other symptoms include:

- Pelvic pain or pressure
- Bleeding or spotting between menstrual periods
- Unusually frequent urination
- Abdominal swelling or discomfort
- Low back or leg pain
- Fatigue or low energy from heavy periods and excessive bleeding
- Constipation
- Repeated miscarriages

Fibroids need estrogen to grow. In perimenopause, estrogen dominance becomes more common and feeds them, causing them to grow larger and potentially exhibit symptoms. However, when estrogen lowers in menopause, they shrink and symptoms subside. That said, it is still possible during menopause to grow fibroids and experience the symptoms of them. Menopausal women with estrogen dominance may not experience a decrease in fibroids, and women taking hormone therapy in perimenopause or menopause won't see a lessening of their symptoms because hormone therapy usually contains estrogen.

There are five types of fibroids, classified by their location.

1. **Intramural:** most common type, embedded in the muscles of the uterus.
2. **Subserosal:** grow on the outside of the uterus; can be large enough to pressure surrounding organs.
3. **Pedunculated:** when a subserosal fibroid grows a stem or slender base that supports the tumor, called a pedicle.
4. **Submucosal:** grow underneath the mucous membrane that lines the uterus, the endometrium. This type is most often the cause of heavy bleeding.
5. **Cervical:** located in the cervix and often accompanied by fibroids in other areas of the uterus. The most common symptom is irregular or heavy bleeding.

Often fibroids are found during a routine pelvic exam, but ultrasound, MRI, hysteroscopy (a slender telescope inserted through the cervix and into the uterus), and laparoscopy (a thin scope inserted through a tiny incision near the navel) can detect fibroids as well.

Heavy Bleeding in Menopause

Once you have reached menopause and have gone twelve consecutive months without a period, you should not experience vaginal bleeding unless you are on hormone therapy. Women taking continuous combined doses of estrogen and a progesterone (both hormones taken daily) may experience spotting to bleeding. Other than that, all vaginal bleeding should stop in menopause. If you are in menopause and still bleeding or spotting, you need to contact your trusted healthcare provider right away to determine the cause. These may include:

Fibroids: Symptoms may persist even after the natural drop in estrogen in menopause; menopause decreases your risk of developing new fibroids and should decrease the size of preexisting fibroids. (See "Spotlight: Fibroids" on page 234 for more.)

Age-related thinning (atrophy) of endometrial tissue: As the tissue lining the uterus thins with age, it may cause bleeding.

Endometrial (or uterine) polyps: These are small, soft benign growths of the uterine lining.

Endometrial hyperplasia: This is an overgrowth of cells lining the uterus, and is considered a precursor to endometrial cancer.

Cancer: Postmenopausal bleeding is a common symptom of endometrial cancer, but it also can be caused by cervical and vulvar cancer.

The most important thing? Don't freak out, or on the flip side, ignore any bleeding. Talk to your trusted healthcare provider about it so you can decide the best next steps.

Why It's Happening

Heavy bleeding during perimenopause is linked to the natural ebb and flow of estrogen and progesterone, but other imbalanced hormones and the root causes driving them can make it worse by contributing to estrogen dominance. Getting a handle on these additional factors such as stress and gut and liver issues will help reduce bleeding and fibroids.

As mentioned, there are other reasons you may experience heavy bleeding. Work with your trusted healthcare provider to rule out pregnancy-related issues, polyps, infection, and other possibilities.

Wild Hormone Fluctuations

You've heard it before, but you just can't underestimate the impact of the unpredictable hormonal roller-coaster ride that is perimenopause. By our late thirties to early forties, our ovaries are on the downswing, and the once-predictable rise and fall of estrogen and progesterone associated with our menstrual cycle becomes unpredictable. Estrogen production becomes erratic, spiking and crashing in a last-ditch effort by the body to support a pregnancy. Meanwhile, fewer ovulations mean lower progesterone. When these two dance partners are out of sync, we can experience a range of symptoms, including heavy bleeding. And this is completely normal.

Estrogen Dominance

Declining progesterone during perimenopause means insufficient progesterone to oppose estrogen, especially the more aggressive type of estrogen, estradiol (E2). This imbalance is called estrogen dominance. And voilà: irregular bleeding, including heavier-than-normal flow.

Declining progesterone isn't the only reason for estrogen dominance, though. Your liver is responsible for breaking down used-up estrogen and helping to eliminate it safely from the body. A sluggish liver with less-than-stellar detoxification capabilities won't be able to metabolize estrogen correctly. Instead of estrogen leaving the body, it recirculates throughout, contributing to high estrogen levels and estrogen dominance (see Sluggish Liver in this chapter for more detail on how the liver breaks down estrogen).

And we can't forget about the gut. A special kind of bacteria living in our gut microbiome, the estrobolome, helps break down estrogen even further after it's been processed by the liver. If too many "bad" bacteria proliferate in the estrobolome, they can undo all of the work the liver has done to deactivate estrogen and reactivate it, sending estrogen right back into the bloodstream. This is why a healthy gut microbiome is so important for regulating estrogen levels.

Finally, xenoestrogens, those man-made chemicals that act as endocrine disruptors and have an estrogen-like effect on the body, are big-time contributors to estrogen dominance.

Stress

Yup, more stress means more flow. Chronic stress is one of the main drivers of estrogen dominance and its symptoms, including heavy bleeding. When your stress response is activated often and over extended periods of time, your body prioritizes making cortisol, your "stress" hormone. Unfortunately, that means progesterone production gets hijacked. You see, both cortisol and progesterone are made from pregnenolone, and when your body favors making cortisol, less progesterone is produced, leaving a low supply to offset estrogen.

Genetic Predisposition

Our genes play a role in our ability to metabolize estrogen, and some of us may have a predisposition, or a genetic single nucleotide polymorphism (SNP; pronounced "snip"), that can make it more likely for us to have estrogen dominance and experience its symptoms, such as heavy bleeding. Remember, genes are not destiny! Just because you have a genetic predisposition doesn't mean you're destined to struggle with estrogen dominance. And just because your DNA test came back indicating a predisposition does not mean you need to spring into action. We now know that lifestyle plays a major role in how genes turn on and off, giving you a lot of input into how your genes express themselves.

The two genes—both of which you can get tested for—that influence your ability to break down estrogen are:

COMT. The COMT gene codes for the COMT enzyme, which helps you break down neurotransmitters such as dopamine, epinephrine, norepinephrine, and estrogen. A SNP on this gene can slow down this enzyme, taking longer to remove excess estrogen, contributing to estrogen dominance.

MTHFR. A SNP on the MTHFR gene makes it difficult for the body to perform a process critical for estrogen detoxification: methylation. Methylation is essential for many significant biochemical reactions in the body that regulate the activity of your cardiovascular, reproductive, neurological, and detoxification systems. When the MTHFR gene is mutated, the methylation process does not work efficiently. A lack of methylation means estrogens are recirculated instead of eliminated, elevating estrogen levels and bringing on estrogen dominance.

Sluggish Liver

If your flow is on the heavy side, it's time to give your liver some TLC and support its ability to detoxify estrogen. In two phases, the liver works hard to remove estrogens safely, and there are several ways the process can go sideways.

In Phase 1 of the process, known as oxidation, estrogen enters the liver and is broken down into smaller pieces called estrogen metabolites. There are three main types: 2-OH, 4-OH, and 16-OH. Some metabolites are better than others. 2-OH is considered a "good" one, helping to prevent symptoms of estrogen dominance and estrogen-based cancers and even acting as an antioxidant. 4-OH and 16-OH are considered the "bad" ones. 4-OH may increase your risk for estrogen-based cancers and 16-OH causes cells to proliferate or grow, causing symptoms like breast tenderness, fibroids, and thickened uterine lining causing heavy periods and clots.

We want to promote 2-OH metabolites during Phase 1. What can inhibit that conversion? Nutritional deficiency, toxic exposure, alcohol consumption, low protein intake, and medications such as acetaminophen (brand name Tylenol).

The metabolites produced in Phase 1 are more toxic than the estrogen that originally entered the liver, so it's important to move them along through Phase 1 and into Phase 2 as efficiently as possible. We don't want these toxic metabolites hanging around!

In Phase 2, also known as conjugation, your liver neutralizes the 2-OH and 4-OH metabolites. The healthiest way to neutralize 2-OH and 4-OH estrogen metabolites is through a process called methylation so they can be excreted in bile, urine, or stool. Phase 2 can go awry if we lack the nutrients needed to pair with the estrogen metabolites.

To go as planned, both phases rely on a healthy liver and vital nutrients. Any deficiency means harmful metabolites and too much estrogen back in our bloodstream.

Gut Issues

If you read about how a sluggish liver is a root cause of estrogen dominance and heavy bleeding, you know that that estrogen is broken down in Phase 1 of the liver detoxification process and neutralized in Phase 2. Guess what? There's a Phase 3! It's time to get that estrogen gone from your body, and this is where your gut comes in. Neutralized estrogen metabolites can go to your kidneys and then out of your body either through your bladder and urine or with your bile into your small intestine and through the rest of your gut for elimination in your stool.

By the time estrogen is in the gut, it's in a package with a bow ready to get pooped out. But before it leaves your body, it has to pass through your gut microbiome and the special collection of bacteria, the estrobolome, that handle estrogen excretion. If those bacteria are out of balance, they can reactivate the neutralized estrogen and send it back into circulation, basically nullifying everything the liver worked so hard to do. Hello, estrogen dominance! Maintaining a healthy gut microbiome through proper diet, including probiotics and fermented foods, will keep neutralized estrogen moving along and prevent reabsorption.

And we need to keep things moving along by supporting our gut health to have regular bowel movements. Constipation makes estrogen dominance worse by hindering the final flush of estrogen out of our system. Proper hydration will help to keep your body regular, as will lots of healthy fiber.

Thyroid Issues

Hypothyroidism, or an underactive thyroid, is a frequent cause of menstrual irregularities, including heavy periods. Without sufficient thyroid hormone, you may not make enough progesterone or the estrogen-binding protein SHBG, both of which contribute to estrogen dominance. Low thyroid function also hinders the liver and gut's estrogen detoxing powers, further increasing your estrogen load.

Hyperthyroidism, or an overactive thyroid, usually results in infrequent or missed periods with shorter, lighter flow.

What You Can Do to Relieve Heavy Bleeding and Fibroids

There are tons of natural options to lighten your flow, ease fibroids symptoms, and reverse estrogen dominance. While essential oils can't cure or heal any of your heavy bleeding or fibroid issues, they can support the hormones that affect them and help alleviate the resulting symptoms. Each of the oils in my top five list supports your body in finding its own equilibrium. I recommend trying each to figure out which ones work the best for you and experimenting to see which combinations support your body's needs the most.

Use these in concert with the Hormone Makeover Program in Part III to find a better balance between estrogen and progesterone and support liver and gut estrogen detoxification. Also turn to the chapters on stress and digestive issues for more help targeting those root causes.

If you've tried the natural approach and still need more assistance, check out the additional options for heavy bleeding and fibroids at the end of this chapter. Always work with your trusted healthcare provider to find the best way forward for you and your unique situation and to rule out more serious medical causes of heavy bleeding.

Top 5 Essential Oils to Relieve Heavy Bleeding and Fibroids

1. Clary Sage
2. Lavender
3. Copaiba
4. Frankincense
5. Yarrow/Pom

Essential Oil Blends

Diffuser Blends

Hormonal Balance Diffuser Blend

2 drops Clary Sage essential oil
2 drops Lavender essential oil
I drop Ylang Ylang essential oil

Unwind Diffuser Blend

4 drops Bergamot essential oil
2 drops Frankincense essential oil

Boost and Balance Diffuser Blend

3 drops Clary Sage essential oil
3 drops Bergamot essential oil

Rollerball Blends

Menstrual Support Rollerball Blend

8 drops Clary Sage essential oil
6 drops Lavender essential oil
4 drops Geranium essential oil
4 drops Copaiba essential oil
Carrier oil of your choice

Roll on your abdomen and pulse points prior to and during menstruation.

Pelvic Soothe Rollerball Blend

8 drops Clary Sage essential oil
6 drops Lavender essential oil
5 drops Frankincense essential oil
5 drops Copaiba essential oil

5 drops Peppermint essential oil

Carrier oil of your choice

Roll on your abdomen and gently massage to ease pain and cramping.

Love Your Liver Rollerball Blend

5 drops Geranium essential oil

5 drops Frankincense essential oil

3 drops Ginger essential oil

3 drops Grapefruit essential oil

2 drops Rosemary essential oil

Carrier oil of your choice

Roll over your liver to support natural detox and healthy endocrine function.

Slow the Flow Rollerball Blend

8 drops Clary Sage essential oil

6 drops Lavender essential oil

4 drops Clove essential oil

4 drops Yarrow/Pom essential oil

Carrier oil of your choice

Roll on your abdomen and massage in slowly to reduce the symptoms associated with menorrhagia.

Supplements and Herbal Remedies to Relieve Heavy Bleeding and Fibroids

Reversing estrogen dominance is the best way to ease heavy bleeding and fibroids. These supplements and herbs are some of my favorites to restore estrogen and progesterone to balance and support your gut and liver for healthy estrogen detoxification, while reducing inflammation and alleviating pain. Consider these in addition to the supplements I recommend as part of the 21-Day Makeover Plan (page 272).

Supplements

ESSENTIALLY WHOLE® HORMONE BALANCE

Hormone Balance is my own formulation of hormone-loving ingredients in one convenient package. It contains powerful ingredients such as black cohosh, chaste tree, DIM, calcium, magnesium, B-complex vitamins, and more that all contribute to healthy uterine and menstrual health. They are also essential to relieve estrogen dominance by ensuring your body is able to detoxify itself of excess estrogens.

IRON (30-100 MG/DAY)

If you have been bleeding heavily during your period for any length of time, it is highly likely that you are deficient in iron. When you don't have enough iron, your tissues won't get all the oxygen they need. Symptoms of deficiency include fatigue, headaches, shortness of breath, paleness, and even anxiety.

VITAMIN C (1,000–3,000 MG/DAY)

Vitamin C is a natural anti-inflammatory to help ease your heavy bleeding and the pain that comes along with it. It is also necessary to help your body absorb iron, so you should always take vitamin C at the same time as your iron supplement.

DIM (DIINDOLYMETHANE) (100 MG/DAY)

DIM, a compound found in cruciferous vegetables, shows great promise for its ability to increase the body's production of healthy estrogen while decreasing the bad. DIM supplements can alleviate symptoms of PMS and help reduce your heavy bleeding, because of its phytonutrient and antioxidant compounds. Check out your source of DIM before you start taking it to be sure you're getting only the best ingredients. I recommend Essentially Whole® DIM Complete because

I know it has been formulated with only the purest ingredients to get your body what it needs!

Herbs

CHASTEBERRY (*VITEX AGNUS-CASTUS*) (150–250 MG/DAY)

Chasteberry (or vitex, or chaste tree) is a well-recognized herbal supplement to treat menstrual issues and PMS. Chasteberry can increase the progesterone levels in your body to help you combat symptoms of estrogen dominance and regulate your bleeding.

GINGER (2 CAPSULES OF DRIED GINGER [1G/CAPSULE] TWICE/DAY)

Studies show that ginger supplementation is as effective as over-the-counter and some prescription pain relievers for painful cramping, while also helping to ease bloating and heavy bleeding during your period. You can expect to see the effects of ginger within three cycles of beginning the supplement.

RESVERATROL (150–450 MG/DAY)

Resveratrol is a powerful polyphenol compound that shows great promise for optimizing your uterine health. In particular, it can shrink and prevent the growth of fibroids by keeping your uterine cells healthy due to its strong antioxidant and regulatory properties.

DONG QUAI (500 MG UP TO 6 TIMES/DAY)

Dong quai is an ancient Chinese herb that acts as a phytoestrogen in your body. Essentially, it can take the place of the hormone estrogen when you aren't producing enough of it so you can achieve optimal balance for your body. It is also recognized for its benefits for menstrual regulation while calming heavy bleeding by helping your uterine muscles to relax.

CURCUMIN (200–500 MG, TWICE/DAY)

Found in the rich, yellow Indian spice turmeric, curcumin has a host of anti-inflammatory health benefits for your body. Reducing inflammation can help with your symptoms of estrogen dominance, as well as reducing the amount of pain and bleeding that comes with your menstrual cycle.

Dr. Mariza's Hormone-Loving Rituals and Protocols

Castor Oil Pack Ritual

Derived from the castor oil plant *Ricinus communis*, castor oil has been used for centuries to support healing, especially in the reproductive system. Promoting ovarian, uterine, and fallopian tube health, castor oil stimulates the lymphatic and circulatory system, allowing for the removal of waste and toxins from the pelvis. Many women have found that castor oil packs provide relief from endometriosis pain, menstrual cramps, and other pelvic issues. Though castor oil packs can increase bleeding, I suggest trying them, as they may be what you need to release thick clots and heavy flow. I recommend applying the Pelvic Soothe Rollerball Blend (page 242) before applying your castor oil pack once each week. Use a castor oil pack with a hot water bottle on top for two to three hours or wear overnight. Check out the Resources section for where to buy my favorite pack.

Additional Treatment Options for Heavy Bleeding

Work with your doctor to figure out the root cause so you can tailor your treatment. If you find that you need more support after trying more natural options, consider the following.

NSAIDs

Nonsteroidal anti-inflammatory drugs such as ibuprofen, aspirin, and naproxen can effectively reduce both blood loss and painful cramping. Be mindful with NSAIDs, as they burden the gut and liver.

Bioidentical Progesterone Cream, 2% strength

Due to decreased progesterone levels, I recommend supplementing with a natural progesterone cream to counteract estrogen dominance and potentially decrease heavy bleeding, fibrocycstic breasts and loss of sex drive. The body absorbs the cream well, making it more bio-available than progesterone pills, which need to first be broken down by the liver. I typically recommend 20 mg (1/4 teaspoon) rubbed into your hands, inner arms, stomach, and thighs two times per day for three weeks on and one week off (during your period). If your period is irregular, try to time your week off when your period occurs.

Birth Control Pill

Low-estrogen birth control pills can help ease heavy, irregular periods, but I recommend opting for the lowest effective dose for the shortest amount of time.

That said, it's an all-too-common practice for women in perimenopause to be encouraged to go on the pill as a way of easing the symptoms. There are a few serious considerations to keep in mind. You will be discouraged from taking birth control pills if you are a forty-plus-year-old woman who is obese, smokes cigarettes, or has migraine headaches, high blood pressure, or diabetes. Like all hormonal contraceptives, the pill comes with serious risks, including blood clots, cardiovascular disease, and venous thromboembolism (a blood clot that starts in a vein).

Another huge consideration is the fact that you won't know if you've entered menopause because the synthetic hormones in birth control pills mask your body's natural hormonal changes and even causes side effects that are similar to menopause symptoms. You'll have to come off the pill to know if you've had your last menstrual period and reached menopause, which is why I recommend a short stint. Risks increase if you take the pill during menopause, adding synthetic hormones into the natural changes occurring in your body.

Bottom line: If you are currently on the pill, I recommend having a conversation with your trusted healthcare provider about getting off it. Otherwise, how will you know what is normal for your body? The pill is a contraceptive, not a long-term solution to hormone imbalance.

Dilation and Curettage (D&C)

This surgical treatment for heavy bleeding involves scraping the lining of the uterus and removing excess tissue. It is normally used after a miscarriage, but some doctors may recommend it as a solution for heavy bleeding or perform it prior to an endometrial ablation.

Endometrial Ablation

This procedure destroys the lining of the uterus (the endometrium) to decrease or completely stop bleeding. Endometrial ablation does not shrink fibroids but can reduce the heavy bleeding caused by them. It should be done only if you don't want to get pregnant, because removing the uterine lining removes the place for the fertilized egg to implant. Pregnancies that occur after an endometrial ablation have an increased risk of miscarriage and other serious complications. There are several different types of endometrial ablation depending on the instrument used:

- **Hydrothermal:** Fluid is pumped into the uterus and heated to destroy the uterine lining.
- **Balloon therapy:** A specially designed balloon is inserted into the uterus through a tube and filled with heated fluid. As the balloon expands, it destroys the uterine lining.
- **High-energy radio waves:** Radio waves are used to heat up and destroy the uterine lining.
- **Freezing:** Also known as cryoablation, an instrument with a cold tip freezes the uterus to destroy the lining.
- **Microwave:** Microwaves are passed through the uterus to destroy the uterine lining.

A partial endometrial ablation (PEA) ablates or destroys only the anterior or posterior uterine lining instead of the whole thing. If this is recommended for you by a trusted healthcare provider, I recommend the NovaSure procedure as the safest form, using radio-frequency energy through netting.

Additional Treatment Options for Fibroids

Fibroids will respond to the approaches listed below. Keep in mind that unless they are impacting the normal functioning of your life or causing anemia, fibroids don't necessarily need to be treated at all. In many cases, fibroids don't cause adverse health consequences or symptoms; you can live with them. For this reason, doctors often embrace the "wait and watch" mindset when it comes to fibroids that are not causing any harm. If you're close to menopause, you may want to wait and see what happens when your estrogen levels drop and your fibroids will likely shrink on their own.

Birth Control Pill

The pill won't eliminate or shrink your fibroids but can help manage your symptoms, such as pain and heavy bleeding. See the Birth Control Pill entry under Additional Treatment Options for Heavy Bleeding above.

Depo-Provera

Depo-Provera is the brand name for medroxyprogesterone acetate, a form of hormonal birth control. This long-lasting injection of progestin, the synthetic form of progesterone, may shrink fibroids and lighten flow. It should be considered a quick emergency option due to severe heavy bleeding and anemia.

Gonadotropin-Releasing Hormone (GnRH) Agonists

Gonadotropin-releasing hormone (GnRH) agonists block the production of estrogen, shrinking and stopping the growth of fibroids. They put you in a temporary menopause-like state complete with all of the usual symptoms: hot flashes, vaginal dryness, and sleep issues. For this reason, GnRH agonists are rarely used for more than six months. Also, long-term use is associated with bone loss. Fibroids usually grow back once you stop taking the drug, so GnRH agonists are best used as a short-term solution, a bridge to menopause, or before surgery to shrink fibroids.

Acessa Procedure

A minimally invasive, uterine-sparing solution for women with fibroids. It uses radio waves to destroy each fibroid without damaging surrounding tissues.

Endometrial Ablation

An option for heavy bleeding due to submucosal fibroids. This procedure destroys the lining of the uterus, known as the endometrium, to
reduce bleeding. It can be done in several ways—for example, using
heat or cold. See the Endometrial Ablation entry under Additional
Treatment Options for Heavy Bleeding above for more information.

Uterine Artery Embolization (UAE)

In this minimally invasive procedure, also called uterine fibroid em-
bolization, the blood supply to the fibroids is blocked, causing them to
shrink and reduce bleeding.

Myomectomy

This surgical procedure removes fibroids while keeping the uterus in
place. Several techniques are available depending on the size and location of the fibroid. For example, if the fibroid is small and inside the
uterus, the surgery can be done with a hysteroscope or a thin, lighted
tube. Many or very large fibroids growing in the uterine wall will most
likely be removed through an incision in your lower belly, an abdominal
myomectomy. During laparoscopic surgery, a smaller incision is made.

Hysterectomy

A hysterectomy is a surgical procedure to remove the uterus and all
of the attached fibroids. Approximately 600,000 hysterectomies are
performed in the United States each year—the highest hysterectomy
rate in the industrialized world—and nearly all of them are elective.
Most, some estimate 90 percent, aren't necessary; women could have
been treated in ways that preserved the uterus.

There are three types of hysterectomy:

- **Total.** In this surgery, generally for large, widespread fibroid
  clusters, the entire uterus and cervix are removed.

- **Partial/subtotal.** With this surgery, only your upper uterus is removed.
- **Radical.** The most extensive form of hysterectomy removes your uterus, upper vagina, cervix, and parametria (surrounding tissues of the uterus and vagina). It is mostly used to treat certain gynecological cancers and rarely used for fibroids.

A hysterectomy is major surgery and a permanent solution for severe fibroids and bleeding after all other less invasive approaches have been tried first. The removal of the uterus means you will stop getting your period and cannot get pregnant. If both of your ovaries are removed as well, you may immediately enter menopause (called surgical menopause). In addition to the short-term risks associated with the surgery, such as blood clots and infection, studies have shown potential long-term health issues, so be sure to discuss the risks with your trusted healthcare provider.

Is a Hysterectomy for Fibroids Right for You?

Hysterectomy is one of the most common gynecological surgeries, yet so many women don't really understand the procedure, the impact it will have on their body, or the alternatives for treating fibroids. A 2017 survey commissioned by the Society of Interventional Radiology found that 20 percent of the women surveyed believe hysterectomy was the only treatment for uterine fibroids and 19 percent believed fibroids were cancerous and required the removal of the uterus. No and no! You have an array of less radical options (and fibroids are not cancerous). A hysterectomy for heavy bleeding and fibroids should be the solution of last resort.

Before you decide a hysterectomy is the best option for you, have you:

- Tried all of the natural options available?
- Explored other nonsurgical and surgical options?
- Investigated and spoken with your trusted healthcare provider about the risks and side effects of the procedure?
- Decided that the symptoms are affecting your quality of life significantly enough to outweigh the risks and side effects of the surgery?
- Determined that you do not want to have children?
- Considered that you may experience menopausal symptoms after the surgery?
- Discussed the sexual side effects and risks?
- Reviewed the potential long-term health risks, such as high blood, obesity, and heart disease?

PART III

The 21-Day Hormone Makeover Program

Chapter 15

Get Ready: Welcome to the 21-Day Hormone Makeover Program

This is it—the time to redefine your midlife and embrace your future with grace and joy. Welcome to my 21-Day Hormone Makeover Program!

Spending the first part of your life giving everything that you have to everyone around you not only blessed your life, but allowed your health and your inner self to slide into second place. And I understand that: All women do! I have learned the hard way that being burned out is not a badge of honor. Burnout won't help us reach our goals faster or create a life filled with loving relationships. As you have probably learned, when you are burned out, it's practically impossible to show up for the people and projects that matter. And if we fulfill our dreams or goals, it's difficult to celebrate those moments.

But today, in this modern world full of natural healing possibilities, *you* get to redefine what midlife looks like for you. Right now *you* get to decide how you want to feel, look, and be for the world.

The Three A's: Accept, Anticipate, and Adapt

You deserve to be honored, cherished, and respected as you transition into this part of your life. I encourage you to follow the mantra that has worked for so many women I have helped: accept, anticipate, and adapt.

Accept that changes to your body are coming. You've already read a good chunk of this book and have empowered yourself with knowledge. You have the power of science on your side because you understand what's going on in your body and the hormonal fluxes that will influence this next phase. But now you also know that there are several other factors or root causes impacting your health, and they are influenced by lifestyle choices over which you have a lot of control. Proper nutrition will nourish your body, essential oils will bridge the gaps for sustainable health, and tailored high-quality supplementation will support your cellular function from the inside out.

Anticipate these changes by giving yourself the love and self-care that you deserve. Honor your body and marvel at the amazing job it has done so far in your life. The fact that you are reading these words right now shows me that you are already anticipating what is to come and are eager to provide your body with the foundational lifestyle changes that it so craves and needs at this pivotal point in your life. Know that your body is ripe for healing miracles!

Adapt your current routines and lifestyle based on your needs, now that you have a deeper understanding of how your body works and understand how to look out for key signs and symptoms. The 21-Day Hormone Makeover Program is carefully choreographed and designed to address your individual needs. The plan itself is adaptable based on your biggest area of focus. No one plan will look the same, so please find joy in selecting the rituals, routines, protocols, and delicious meals to serve your body. By securing your foundational health and putting rituals and routines into place, you will set yourself up for lasting success. Get ready to saunter into the future with ease and grace, knowing that you have done the work and set the tone of more energy and joy.

Anchor Your Success

Success in this program depends on you and the choices that you make. But having guided thousands of women to their own personal success, I have discovered that game-changing results rely on three anchors: accountability, commitment, and vision. These are three small hinges that will help open that big door to the rest of your life.

Accountability

Speed-dial your bestie and tell her your plan. Ask for her help, or better yet, invite her to join you. Who doesn't love an accountability buddy? Do your best to anticipate what you think might be the most difficult thing for you in the program, and specifically ask for their help with that. If movement seems daunting, invite them to exercise with you. If the meal plan seems scary, invite them to meal prep with you. No matter how little, no matter how large, your bestie or family member can help you create success. There is nothing like a tandem effort and loving accountability.

Commitment

There is no soft start to this program—you gotta commit and get going! Set a start date, do your prep work, and take the first step into the rest of your life. This program is intentionally flexible for each woman to take the reins of her own future, but there is one firm step: Do It. You have to love yourself enough to commit and take the first step. That is where having an accountability partner will help, and having a vision will guide you.

Vision

Women who have the most success in this program have a clear vision of what they want to be or see in the future. My mom knew that she wanted to experience more energy again, to feel in control of her own health and to enjoy playing tennis with her friends after work. But most of all, she wanted to feel at home in her own body. I have a feeling that her vision probably resonates with how you are feeling right now, but you are a unique woman. So, let's set an intention for how you would love to feel. Let's peer into your future and hold the vision of the woman you are going to become. Complete the vision exercise below to discover the woman waiting to greet you 22 days from now at the end of the program.

Create a Vision for Your Success

With a clear vision for how you want to feel at the end of the 21-Day Hormone Makeover Program, you instantly create an anchor to hold you steady when times get tough and you feel like you want to quit. When creating your vision, focus on what you would love to have in your life and what you want for yourself. Write, in vivid detail, about your health accomplishments and epic wins. Allow yourself to dream big and be specific. This detailed vision of who you will become is much more than an anchor; it's a launch pad to your future healthy and youthful self. It's that powerful!

The key is to put your vision into words in your journal or on a piece of paper, and then revisit your vision every morning for a few minutes before you start your day.

Step 1: Grab your journal or a piece of paper.

Step 2: Write this down: It's Day 22 and I have completed the 21-Day Hormone Makeover Program. It all worked out for me! I am grateful and thankful that I feel . . . Finish that sentence and write several others with the vision you are holding for yourself. Remember to be specific and detailed.

Step 3: When you've finished, unlock your full vision potential by ending with this abundance amplifier, a statement that opens the door for endless wins: *And all of this or something even better still!*

Step 4: Sign your name as a commitment to yourself and read it every day during the program.

Did you love this exercise? Or did it stretch you to write out a vision for yourself? Or both? When I did this exercise for the first time it was a challenge because I was still holding on to limiting beliefs about my worth and I didn't believe that I deserved to have a vision for myself. I didn't believe it was appropriate to ask myself, "What would I love?" But I did it anyway and my entire life changed. That's why I am excited to give you this beautiful vision gift. If you want to dive even deeper and create a vision for your life, check out the link to the *Vision Vortex Guide* created by my bestie, Jennifer Hudye, in the Resources section on page 358.

The Science Behind Your Success

To create this program, I've leveraged scientific research with the power of nature to support and heal your body by resetting your gut, liver, and stress. Targeting these three addresses the root causes of your symptoms head on, balancing your hormones and restoring your energy and joy.

The Hormone-Balancing Trifecta: Gut, Liver, and Stress Reset

The key to your success is giving love to your gut and liver, and resetting your stress response. All three help to rebalance your metabolism, support your thyroid and adrenal function, and stabilize your mood. Healing this hormone-balancing trifecta is integrated into every recipe, every remedy, every essential oil protocol, every self-care routine. Here's how each works to reset and rebalance, allowing your body to heal itself.

#1 Gut Reset: Reestablishing a Healthy Microbiome

A healthy gut depends on a balanced microbiome. Promoting balance in your microbiome and removing inflammation is a central component in the plan that I have carefully crafted for you. By focusing on your digestion, you can optimize your hormones and your energy levels at the same time. Even if you are thinking, "I don't have a gut issue; it's my hormones!" I invite you to trust me that your digestive function is playing a much bigger role than you think.

#2 Liver Reset: Restoring Healthy Liver Function

Responsible for metabolizing, regulating, and detoxifying hormones in the body, your liver performs more than 500 vital functions for your body, filtering over a liter of your blood every minute of every day, converting vitamins to active forms and storing them for later use, controlling blood sugar, signaling satiety, and so much more. An overburdened liver means estrogen dominance and a high toxic load. This is why your liver always needs love!

In the Hormone Makeover Program, you will be focusing on liver-loving foods that aid with liver detoxification as well as gut elimination. These foods are all on the Yes foods list and built into your meal plan and recipes. Some of my personal favorites are: avocado, leafy greens, fresh herbs, garlic, broccoli, and cauliflower.

#3 Stress Reset: Reducing Unhealthy Stress Patterns

Chronic stress is the most common root cause of hormone imbalance, exhaustion, brain fog, and even stubborn belly fat. I believe that stress is one of the major drivers for perimenopause and menopause symptoms.

Reducing our daily stress and calming our stress-response system, the HPA axis, is imperative to feeling our best and giving our body a break. We will do this through self-care rituals supported by the healing power of essential oils, high-quality supplements designed to restore balance to your body, and the 21-Day Meal Plan, which focuses on hormone-loving nutrition.

Foundational Lifestyle Rituals

The entire 21-Day Hormone Makeover Program was designed to help you improve your whole self, from inside out and outside in. It focuses on positive choices that you can make to change your journey while strengthening the gut-liver-stress trifecta. In order for you to have the best success possible on the program, you cannot ignore the bedrock that grounds your body's overall functioning. After helping thousands of women—my mom included—to regain energy and vitality and thrive in peri/menopause, I realized those who have the most success on this program are the women who commit to strengthening their foundation. These foundational lifestyle rituals are the ground floor, the basic support that your body needs to function each and every day.

Foundational Support #1: Hormone-Loving Nutrition

The easiest component of this program is the hormone-loving nutrition, because you can simply follow the recipes on the meal plan I have laid out for you. Where it gets individual is the option to make substitutions and swaps based on what you like. While I encourage you to try some new flavors because I have personally tested and love *every* recipe in this book, it's okay for you to create your own meals as long as you follow the Yes/No food lists.

Food affects every cell in your body, and your choices can move you closer, or further away, from inflammation. Certain choices contribute to inflammation, insulin resistance, blood sugar instability, and more driving factors that are behind your weight gain, estrogen dominance, and uncomfortable peri/menopausal symptoms. Choosing foods that fight against this trend is going to be your ticket to reclaiming the life you've been missing.

As you walk through the 21-Day Program, I want you to feel successful along the way. That's why in the coming chapters, I have broken down more targeted ways you can address your gut, liver, thyroid, adrenals, and blood sugar balance complete with high-quality supplementation protocols so you can personalize the plan to fit your needs.

Foundational Support #2: Move Your Body!

Moving your body is a nonnegotiable need that we all have. While the specific activity can be based on your preferences, daily movement must be an integral part of your journey. You've got to get that body stretched and moving for cardiovascular health, cellular vitality, muscular support, and to maintain your metabolism.

You may have noticed that I haven't said the word "exercise" yet. That's because there are too many negative connotations with exercise, making it a chore and not a joy. Only you know the kind of movement your body needs and what it will respond to overall!

This is the movement mindset that we need to establish for you as an individual. You choose what honors your body and brings you joy. Throughout this book, I have recommended getting outside into nature and mindfully walking because it satisfies a number of needs: stress relief, vitamin D from the sun, movement, and mindfulness. That is a great place to start if you have been sedentary up until now. If you already have a workout routine that you love, then stick to it! Wherever you find yourself before the 21-Day Program, now is a great time to reevaluate and find what movement routine will serve your vision.

Before you begin any new program of movement, it is important that you check with your healthcare provider to ensure your safe participation. If you have a history of heart disease, diabetes, or any other serious health condition, or if you have been sedentary for a year or more, a sudden increase in exercise intensity may put you at a greater risk for complications, so you may need to begin at a much lower intensity and work your way up slowly.

In case you don't know where to start, use the following beginner's guide to develop your own movement routine:

Monday—Strength training, HIIT, or any cardio (heart-pumping) activity

Tuesday—Yoga/stretching with a 10-minute nature walk

Wednesday—30-minute walk/hike/swim and yoga

Thursday—Strength training, HIIT, or any cardio (heart-pumping) activity

Friday—Yoga/stretching with a 10-minute nature walk

Saturday— 30-minute bike/hike/swim and yoga

Sunday—Rest day (nature walk, or yoga/stretching)

No matter what you do, the goal is to get moving. Whether it's a dance party in your kitchen, a hike through the mountains, or a half-marathon (Go for it Mom!), the goal is to support your foundation with what brings you joy.

Foundational Support #3: Daily Self-Care Supported by Essential Oils

Let me walk you through the basics of balancing your day with self-care. There are four parts: a morning ritual, a midday ritual, a night-time ritual, and your Daily Self-Care Journal.

Morning Ritual. Your self-care routine is all about setting the tone for your day! Each day we get to choose the day that we are going to have, and morning rituals really allow that to come into reality. If you wake without a morning routine, you will be subject to a random speed, depending on your coffee intake and blood sugar level. Set your body and mind for success in the morning with rituals that will support you throughout the day, especially when you have a lot on your plate. I shared my favorite Morning Ritual in Chapter 4 on page 87 to give you an example of how to uplift your mind and body with self-love, gratitude, and intention. Select a few of the practices and see what resonates with you. Ask yourself, "What makes my soul sing in the morning?"

Morning Ritual Focus!

The moment I wake up, I'm diffusing my favorite Get Up and Go Blend to help me rock my morning.

Get Up and Go Diffuser Blend

3 drops Wild Orange essential oil

3 drops Peppermint essential oil

Midday Ritual. Midday rituals keep stress at bay. Check out my Midday Stress-Busting Rituals on page 91, incorporating essential oil support, hydration, and mindfulness meditation/prayer. The symptom-based rituals in the chapters of Part II offer other ways to create balance in the middle of your day. Target the symptoms that challenge you the most and use the rituals from those chapters to support you.

Nighttime Ritual. Powering down from your day is just as important as your morning routine. Look over the Nighttime Ritual on page 106 and find some practices that appeal to you. Also, be sure to read over the sleep chapter for powerful routines that support a restful night's sleep. Then try a few to help you de-stress and decompress into your evening. My favorite essential oils are those that support relaxation and sleep, such as Lavender and Roman Chamomile. And if you haven't tried an Epsom Salt Bath Soak, it's high time you indulge! Use the essential oil blends in Chapter 5 for a stress-relieving soak.

Daily Self-Care Journal. You can literally rewire your brain to think positively when you take the time to practice positivity every day, shifting from a negative and stressed mindset to one of gratitude, abundance, confidence, and joy. I created a beautiful journal for myself years ago and you can now get one on my website, but you can also make this activity your own with your own journal. Purchase a blank notebook, something that brings you joy, and choose your favorite pen. Date each page to track your transformation, and then list what you're grateful for and what you want to experience more of that day. Then list your three main self-care rituals for the day. They can be repeated for days or weeks, but I encourage you to start with three each day, even choosing one for the morning, one for midday, and one for evening until you have a repertoire for self-care. Healing foods come next, as you focus on three foods that will nourish your body. Next write down an affirmation that is in alignment with how you want to feel throughout the day. Finally, set your intention for how you will direct your energy for the day; this action plan will be in place when stress, unwanted symptoms, or unpredictable circumstances rock your boat. Then sign it. This is your agreement for the day, your commitment to yourself—a powerful assignation to your positive influence in the world.

Here is a sample from my journal:

Today, June 1, 2020, I am grateful for . . .

1. The sunshine through my windows
2. Breathing in Lavender oil before bed
3. My midday happy playlist
4. Sparkling water with lime and mint
5. My speed-dial bestie—Candace!

Today, I want to experience more laughter instead of anger when things don't go my way.

My 3 Self-Care Rituals for today are . . .

1. Deep Breathing with Superwoman Rollerball Blend
2. Hydrate at the top of every hour (water infusion)
3. Read for 15 mins before I go to bed

I plan to nourish my body with healing foods today . . .

1. Green smoothie with blueberries
2. Avocado in my dinner salad
3. Matcha green tea with almond milk

Daily Affirmation

I am a positive influence on the world.

As I set my intention for today, the most important thing for me to focus on today is . . .

Taking a one-minute break for deep breathing at the top of every hour.

Today, I will follow my inspiration, enjoy myself, and honor my body with self-care rituals and nourishing foods.

X Dr. Mariza Snyder

Foundational Support #4: Reduce Your Toxic Load

Whether you realize it or not, environmental toxins have already invaded your body and threaten your hormone pathways. Research shows that the more bogged down your cells are in resisting foreign chemicals' effects on the body and detoxing them out of your system, the less time they have for supporting your body's overall health. Limiting your exposure while supporting detoxification of your current toxic load is the key to supporting your foundation. The Environmental Working Group's website (ewg.org) is a great resource to assess your current favorite products, and you can learn more about making over your kitchen, cleaning cabinet, personal care products, and medicine cabinet in my book *Smart Mom's Guide to Essential Oils* or following the blog on my website at drmariza.com.

Right now, here are some tips you can do to reclaim control:

- Make over your kitchen by ridding it of processed, chemical-laden foods and plastic storage containers (opt for glass or stainless steel).
- Make over your cleaning cabinet with natural products.
- Make over your personal care products with natural hormone-friendly options.

- Make over your medicine cabinet with the healing power of essential oils.
- Air out your house with open windows for fifty to thirty minutes per day when possible; research shows that the air in your house is more contaminated than that of the environment!
- Run your diffuser with purifying essential oils such as Eucalyptus, Grapefruit, Lemon, and Melaleuca.
- Take off your shoes before entering your house to keep outside contaminants from infiltrating your floors.
- Dust and vacuum regularly.
- Keep oxygen-rich plants inside your home (my favorites are the Peace Lily plant and aloe vera).
- Detox your body from the inside out with consistent hydration, dry brushing, Epsom salt baths, and essential oil support.

Foundational Support #5: Remove Toxic Energy

Toxic energy is just as detrimental to your body as physical toxins, and at this point in your life, it may be time to eliminate unnecessary compromise. It is perfectly okay to say no, and I encourage you to assess your willingness to use this powerful two-letter word. See page 153 for the "Is This Serving Me?" ritual. Energy-draining, toxic people can severely stress you to your core, and if you dread encounters with certain individuals in your life, it is time to say goodbye. Establish boundaries, stand up for your mental health, and create a safe space around you that protects you from energy-sucking vampires.

Unprocessed trauma also adds to the strain on your body and can exacerbate unwanted symptoms. If you haven't done so yet, I encourage you to take time right now to create a Health-Life Timeline (page 37) and see if you can identify a pattern of trauma followed by a health issue. I recommend finding a trusted healthcare provider trained in counseling to help you wade through the waves of emotion that may be causing a storm within. There are also counseling apps that can help you to talk through things with a trained professional. Whatever method you choose, process your trauma and do not let it linger.

Working through past traumas may be the missing piece of your healthcare puzzle!

> ## Instant Energy Protection
>
> Have this blend on hand when toxic energy threatens.
>
> ### Toxic Energy Removal / Energy Protection Rollerball Blend
> 10 drops Lavender essential oil
> 10 drops Bergamot essential oil
> 8 drops Frankincense essential oil
> 4 drops Lemongrass essential oil
> Carrier oil of your choice
>
> *Apply to pulse points, deeply inhale in the aroma, then exhale the negativity.*

Final Steps for Success

As you embark on this incredible transformation, go back to the Create a Vision for Your Success exercise (page 260). What lifestyle areas need firming up to achieve this vision? Are you committed to making this transformation with me? Who do you see coming alongside you as you manifest that vision? Who do you see letting go of during this journey?

Thousands of women have achieved their vision and found the success and symptom relief they desire. I believe you can do it, too. I cannot wait to see your vision manifested on the other side of these 21 days and watch you embrace your future beyond this program.

Chapter 16

Get Set: Prepping for the 21-Day Hormone Makeover Program

Now that you have a clear vision of your success, it's time to prepare for the program. It has ease and flexibility baked in, but I don't want you to sell yourself short by not preparing adequately for the next three weeks. Doing the following prep work will make it that much easier for you to shift your hormones, mood, and overall well-being and fulfill your vision for success.

First, if you haven't already taken my Perimenopause and Menopause Hormone Quiz, do so now (www.drmariza.com/hormonequiz). It'll help you identify specific areas where you may need some extra support. For example, maybe your thyroid or adrenals need an extra dose of love or your insulin levels need to be reset. Or maybe lowering stress and improving mood should be your top priorities.

Your results from the Hormone Quiz will help you anticipate your individual needs and personalize this Makeover Program to fit you. I'm going to break down specific things you can do to target your preferred area. Pick and choose based on what your body is needing during the program.

Next, check off each of the ten prep items listed below before you begin the program.

Preparation

Prep #1 Supplementation

You will experience accelerated results when you have the right supplemental foundation to address nutrient deficiencies. Be sure that you have your supplements on hand before you start the program, as they are an integral component to your success.

You may have already started taking supplements based on my symptom-specific recommendations in Part II. If so, stick with your new regimen and incorporate it with the protocols listed below.

I recommend everyone take the Foundational Daily Hormone Support Protocol, which is carefully formulated and designed for a woman's body at this phase of life. Add additional protocols based on your unique needs from your Perimenopause and Menopause Hormone Quiz results.

If you are not sure which additional protocol you may need, begin by adding the Gut Restore and Liver Restore protocols to the Foundational Daily Hormone Support Protocol. You can always add other protocols later based on the changes that you see once you have firmed up these foundational areas.

While no formal testing is needed before you begin to take these supplements, I do recommend discussing their use with a trusted healthcare provider, especially if you have preexisting health conditions. Trust yourself. Use the knowledge you've gained to support the body you're in now to build the body you see in your vision. In addition to the Essentially Whole® supplements that I specifically formulated and created myself, there are a few other brands that meet my quality specifications reflected in the protocols below. While only you can decide what is best for you, these are the brands that I trust for me and my community—and for you!

Dr. Mariza's Foundational Daily Hormone Support Protocol (for Everyone)

Multivitamin: Designs for Health® Twice Daily MultiTM or Seeking Health® Optimal Multivitamin Methyl One
　Dosage: 1–2 capsules twice a day

These blends contain optimal amounts of many nutrients difficult to obtain through diet alone.

Omega-3 Fish Oil: Nordic Naturals® Ultimate Omega® or Designs for Health® OmegAvail™ Ultra
　Dosage: 1 capsule twice a day with food

Omega-3s help keep down inflammation and prevent damage to your cells, allowing your body to restore balance.

Probiotics: Klaire Labs® Ther-Biotic® Complete; Microbiome Labs MegaSporeBiotic™; or Designs for Health® Probiotic Supreme DF™
　Dosage: 1 capsule twice a day with food

Probiotics are essential for maintaining the health of your gut microbiome, where hormone balance and a strong immune system begin.

Magnesium Bis-Glycinate: Essentially Whole® Magnesium
 Restore or Metagenics® Mag Glycinate
 Dosage: 300-600 mg daily before bed

Magnesium is an essential mineral in your body, and most of us are deficient in it. Having adequate magnesium will help your body rebalance. Essentially Whole® Magnesium Restore also includes magnesium oxide, a form of magnesium shown to relieve hot flashes.

Activated B Vitamins: Essentially Whole® Activated B Complete
 or Thorne® Basic B Complex
 Dosage: 1 capsule daily

B-complex vitamins are essential to keep your brain and body working properly, supporting balance in all of your systems. Always choose an activated, or methylated, form so your body can put the vitamins to use right away.

Gut Restore Add-On Protocol

Gut Repair Nutrients and Herbs: Essentially Whole® Gut Restore
 or GI Revive™ by Designs for Health®
 Dosage: 3 capsules at breakfast; 4 capsules with dinner for 60 days.

These blends combine many amino acids and herbs to support your gut health, restore intestinal integrity, decrease leaky gut, and reduce inflammation.

Comprehensive Digestive Enzymes: Designs for Health®
 Digestzymes™ or Pure Encapsulations® Digestive Enzymes
 Ultra
 Dosage: 1 capsule twice a day with food

Your body naturally produces enzymes to help break down carbs, fats, and proteins, but sometimes it can use a little boost to make sure you have enough and are getting the most nutrition while supporting a healthy microbiome.

Grass-fed Collagen: Bulletproof® Collagen Protein or Vital Proteins® Collagen Peptides

Dosage: 2 tablespoons twice daily (great green smoothie addition)

Collagen restores the integrity of the gut lining and repairs leaky gut.

L-Glutamine: Thorne® Research L-Glutamine Powder or Designs for Health® L-Glutamine Powder

Dosage: 1 teaspoon or 1 scoop daily

L-glutamine is an amino acid that improves the health of your intestinal cells and decreases the permeability of your gut walls to prevent and reverse leaky gut symptoms.

For more gut support recommendations, see Chapter 10, Digestive Issues.

Liver Restore Add-On Protocol

14-Day Liver Detox (Phase 1 and 2 detoxification support): Essentially Whole® 14-Day Detox Kit (includes detox drink packets and liver detox supplements) or Designs for Health® VegeCleanse Plus™ 14-Day Detox Program

Dosage: Follow the instructions on the package.

These detox kits contain nutrients, vitamins, minerals, antioxidants, and hepatics needed to support and balance phase 1 and 2 metabolic pathways and to promote healthy liver function and elimination.

Comprehensive Hormone and Liver Support: Essentially Whole® Hormone Balance or Designs for Health® FemGuard+Balance™

Dosage: 2 capsules twice a day

An ideal blend of herbs, minerals, and nutrients to show your body the love it needs to achieve balanced hormones.

Vitamin C: Essentially Whole® Vitamin C Boost; Liposomal Vitamin C by Designs for Health®; or Seeking Health® Vitamin C Powder
Dosage: I scoop, or I capsule twice daily

Vitamin C is a powerful antioxidant and immune system booster.

Phase 2 Liver Detoxification Support: Essentially Whole® Liver Detox Support or Designs for Health®Detox Antiox™
Dosage: 3 capsules twice daily

These blends are formulated with compounds to support your body's ability to remove toxins from your body through phase II detoxification of the liver.

Sugar/Insulin Balance Add-On Protocol

Myoinositol or D-Chiro-Inositol: Inositol (Powder) by Pure Encapsulations®, or Myo & D-Chiro Inositol by Wholesome Story®
Inositol Powder Dosage: 2 scoops (4.2 g) I–2 times daily
Myo & D-Chiro Inositol Dosage: 2–4 capsules daily

To aid blood sugar balance.

Metabolic Restore: Essentially Whole® Metabolic Restore or Thorne® Research MediBolic®
Dosage: Essentially Whole®: I capsule three times daily with food; Thorne® MediBolic®: 2 scoops with I2–I4 oz water or beverage

These blends provide complete metabolic health support.

Berberine: Thorne® Research Berberine or Klaire Labs® Berberine
Dosage: I capsule two times daily

Berberine is a naturally occurring chemical derived from plants found to combat insulin resistance.

Chromium Picolinate: Thorne® Research Chromium or Designs for Health® Chromium Synergy

   Dosage: 1 capsule daily

The mineral chromium helps insulin work better and improves blood sugar levels.

Vitamin D: Essentially Whole® Vitamin D Complete (with K1 and K2); Vitamin D Synergy™ (with Vitamin K1) by Designs for Health®; or Klaire Labs® Vitamin D Plus K

   Dosage: one capsule daily with food

Note: I recommend getting your levels tested so you can dose appropriately.

Getting enough vitamin D can help reduce insulin resistance and support healthy cell function to get the most energy from the food you eat.

Thyroid Support Add-On Protocol

Vitamin D: Essentially Whole® Vitamin D Complete (with K1 and K2); Vitamin D Synergy™ by Designs for Health®; or Klaire Labs® Vitamin D Plus K

   Dosage: one capsule daily with food

Note: I recommend getting your levels tested so you can dose appropriately.

Many of us are deficient in vitamin D, and studies show that the degree of hypothyroidism is directly connected with vitamin D deficiency.

Thyroid Support Nutrients: Essentially Whole® Thyroid Support or Pure Encapsulations® Thyroid Support Complex

   Dosage: two capsules per day with food

These blends include many of the nutrients your thyroid needs to thrive, helping maintain healthy cortisol levels, processing

blood sugar and insulin in the proper ways, and balancing thyroid conversion levels.

Zinc: Thorne® Research Zinc Picolinate or Klaire Labs® Zinc Plus
    Dosage: one capsule daily with food

Zinc is involved in several steps of thyroid hormone production, regulation, and metabolism.

Adrenal Support Nutrients: Essentially Whole® Adrenal Love or Ortho Molecular Products® Adapten-All
    Dosage: 2 capsules daily with food

A comprehensive blend to provide overall adrenal support.

Selenium: Klaire Labs® Seleno Met™ or Thorne® Research Selenomethionine
    Dosage: one capsule daily with food

Your thyroid requires selenium to metabolize thyroid hormones. Supplementing with selenium helps normalize thyroid function and prevent the start or progression of thyroid diseases.

Iron: Designs for Health® Ferrochel® Iron Chelate or Thorne® Research Ferrasorb®
    Dosage: one capsule daily with food

Your body uses iron to convert the inactive thyroid T4 into active T3.

For more thyroid support recommendations, see Chapter 9, Thyroid Issues.

Adrenal/Stress Recovery Add-On Protocol

Adrenal Support Nutrients: Essentially Whole® Adrenal Love or Ortho Molecular Products ® Adapten-All
    Dosage: 2 capsules daily with food

These blends are formulated with vitamins, amino acids, and adaptogenic herbs to enhance your adrenal glands' function optimally so they don't become overtaxed—and you don't feel the effects of being overly stressed.

Holy Basil: Gaia Herbs® Holy Basil Leaf
> *Dosage:* 1 capsule daily or drink it as a tea

Recognized as "The Queen of Herbs" in Ayurvedic practices, holy basil has a long history of being used to regulate feelings of stress. Users of holy basil experience lessened physical and psychological stress, improved sleep, normalized blood sugar levels, and reduced feelings of exhaustion.

Phosphatidylserine: Klaire Labs® Phosphatidyl Serine or Pure Encapsulations® PS Plus
> *Dosage:* 1 capsule daily with food

A compound that makes up cell membranes and is a major nutrient for the brain, phosphatidylserine helps lower cortisol levels and promotes a healthy stress response.

For more stress and adrenal support recommendations, see Chapter 4, Stress, the Silent Killer.

Mood Balance Add-On Protocol

Vitamin C: Essentially Whole® Vitamin C Boost; Liposomal Vitamin C by Designs for Health®; or Seeking Health® Vitamin C Powder
> *Dosage:* 1 scoop or 1 capsule twice daily

Vitamin C balances mood and reduces anxiety by combating the damage caused to your cells by oxidative stress and clearing toxins.

Gamma-aminobutyric acid (GABA): Essentially Whole® Calm & Restore or Thorne® Research PharmaGABA-100
> *Dosage:* 1–2 capsules daily

GABA (gamma-aminobutyric acid), one of the primary calming neurotransmitters in your body, contributes to so many of your body's processes, including how you handle stress and anxiety, stabilizing your mood, promoting restful sleep, and supporting mental focus while relieving fatigue.

5-HTP: Thorne® Research 5-Hydroxytryptophan, or Bulletproof®
5-HTP

Dosage: 1-2 capsules daily (100–200 mg/day)

Supplementing with 5-HTP, the precursor to the mood-balancing neurotransmitter serotonin, will naturally increase your serotonin levels.

For more mood support recommendations, see Chapter 8, Mood Swings, Anxiety, and Depression.

I am always researching and updating my supplement protocols. Please visit www.drmariza.com/protocols for more hormone-supporting recommendations and protocols.

Prep #2 Kitchen Makeover

The goal is to create a safe place that fosters your success on the 21-Day Program, getting rid of temptations and filling your kitchen with nutritious, hormone-loving foods. It's time to focus your healing with the power of superfoods, healthy fats, protein, and fiber! I encourage anyone living with you to participate in the program, or, at the very least, support you through the program by helping to keep temptations out of plain sight. Here is my two-step kitchen makeover:

#1 Yes/No Clean Out. Using the Yes/No foods lists in Chapter 17, get rid of the No foods. The No foods will sabotage your progress by increasing inflammation, destabilizing blood sugar, and causing hormone chaos.

If you are sharing the kitchen with people who eat food that you are avoiding, consider setting up different areas or shelves in the fridge/freezer/pantry that have clearly defined boundaries so it's easy to keep you on track.

#2 Pantry Restock. Once you have created space for healthy, hormone-loving foods, it's time to take a look at the Meal Plan and the Yes foods list in Chapter 17 and make your shopping list. Get excited, because there are so many delicious options! Don't forget to include pantry basics on your shopping list, such as sea salt, healthy oils and fats, nuts, and spices.

Prep #3 Food Journal

Creating a food journal will help you to both prep meals for your program and record how your body responds to them. Listening to your body will help you identify the foods you can tolerate and the ones that cause inflammatory flare-ups. Be sure to keep track of your digestive patterns, your mood, and any lingering feelings associated with each meal. You can also jot down when you experience food triggers.

Prep #4 Plan Your Meals

The 21-Day Hormone Makeover Meal Plan with Recipes is designed to provide you with easy-to-create meals for breakfast, lunch, and dinner. In addition to recipes, you'll also find a day-by-day meal plan with specific suggestions for each meal of the entire 21-Day Makeover; however, you're not "stuck" with it. If there is a recipe that you don't like, feel free to substitute it with any of the recipes in the plan or replace an ingredient with another healthy option from the Yes foods list.

The most important thing is to plan for your meals so you have the necessary ingredients on hand and aren't scrambling around when you are hangry. That's a setup for a poor choice. Avoid that scenario and take other steps to make nourishing yourself easier. Cook enough food so you have leftovers for lunch or dinner the next day. Make a double of your morning smoothie or shake and have the extra portion for lunch. Or, have a shake or smoothie for dinner. No cooking required!

Prep #5 Essential Oil Support

Select and order the essential oils, diffuser, and supplies (such as glass rollerball bottles) that you plan to use throughout the program, being sure to choose high-quality oils to experience instant wins. Having them on hand makes it easier to use them when you are ready for Day 1.

Prep #6 Buddy System

Get a buddy for your workout sessions or for general support, or invite your bestie to do the program with you. In fact, my husband, Alex, did the meal plan and workouts with me, as well as his own routines. As long as you have someone to support your journey, you are on the right path. It's so much easier to make changes and steps toward health when you're doing it with your friends.

Prep #7 Daily Self-Care Journal

If you haven't purchased one already, I recommend getting a notebook and setting up an example page as I outlined on page 266. Place it in a calm area near your diffuser where you plan to do your Morning Ritual. The more beauty and calm you can bring to your routine, the better!

Prep #8 Hydration

Drinking enough water stabilizes the hunger-signaling hormones, preventing frequent snacking and overeating, and aids the body's detoxification processes. Purchase a stainless steel or glass water bottle that you can take with you throughout the day. In fact, I recommend purchasing two so that you always have one that is clean. Once you embark on the 21-Day Makeover, make it a goal to stay hydrated and mark off your hydration goals each day in your Food Journal.

Prep #9 Schedule Mealtimes

Regular mealtimes help your body get into a routine, cutting down on cravings. My dear friend and emotional eating expert Tricia Nelson calls it Three Meal Magic. If you have to schedule mealtimes into your planner or on your phone, do it. Allow yourself time to eat, to savor, and to allow your body to properly adjust to a three-meals-a-day routine.

Prep #10 Know Your Numbers

Before you begin this program, I invite you to connect with your trusted healthcare provider. Although it's not required to experience success in the program, I believe discussing your symptoms and any health concerns you may have is always a good idea. During your visit, consider getting a few baseline tests done (see The Importance of Testing on page 284) so you can identify areas where you need more support and track your progress. In addition, I encourage you to know your waist-to-hip ratio (WHR) and body mass index (BMI). Oprah says, "Know your numbers," and that has always stuck with me when it comes to measuring for your success.

During this phase in your life it is very important that your personal healthcare practitioner understand and support your specific hormone and menopause symptoms without dismissing, ignoring, or disparaging them. If you feel like you are being dismissed or ignored, it's time to get a second opinion. I have provided some trusted sources to help you find an integrative or functional doctor in the Resources section of this book.

The Importance of Testing

Testing is an important part of discovering hormonal imbalances and root causes in the body. Testing can identify red flags as your hormones fluctuate and even decrease over time. I recommend these preliminary lab tests during perimenopause and menopause. Ask your integrative or functional doctor to order the following:

- A complete blood panel
- Thyroid tests: TSH, Free T3, Free T4, Reverse T3 (RT3), TPOAb, AntiTgAntibody
- DUTCH test (test on days 19–21 of your cycle if you are cycling): Analysis of 35 different hormones: estrogen, progesterone, testosterone, DHEA-S, and cortisol along with their metabolites
- DUTCH oxidative stress marker: 8-hydroxy-2-deoxyguanosine (8-OHdG), melatonin (6-OHMS), and six organic acid tests (OATs) including markers for vitamin B12 (methylmalonate), vitamin B6 (xanthurenate), kynurenate, glutathione (pyroglutamate), dopamine (homovanillate), norepinephrine/epinephrine (vanilmandelate).
- LSH and LH (test on days 2–4 of your cycle if you are cycling)
- Fasting insulin and glucose, glucose tolerance, HDL, and hemoglobin AIC
- IGF-1 (growth hormone)
- 25-hydroxy-vitamin D, vitamin B12, folate
- C-reactive protein (hs-CRP) test

For a complete list of lab tests, test descriptions, and optimal ranges for each test, head over to www.drmariza.com/labtests.

If your doctor won't order these blood tests, order them yourself. Find a list of trusted laboratories in the Resources (page 357).

When you assess the test results, pay attention to the normal ranges. Discuss them with your trusted healthcare provider, and bear in mind that just because your number falls into the "normal" range, that doesn't mean that it's normal for you. Any number at the higher or lower end should be questioned.

Making It a Lifestyle

The heart of this 21-Day Makeover is establishing a series of moments in your day that shift the priority back to you. It's about integrating foods, self-care rituals, movement, essential oils, and supplement protocols that address your unique combination of symptoms to help you reclaim your energy and joy at midlife. Please trust yourself in this process and know that you can find success. Hold on to your Vision for Success as an anchor throughout the entire 21 days. You've got this! Once you start to experience lasting results, you won't ever want to live any other way.

Chapter 17

Go! The 21-Day Hormone Makeover Meal Plan with Recipes

I n order for the Hormone Makeover to be successful, you've got to get real about ending food relationships that have been abusing your body. Throughout your whole life up to this point, you've (mostly) subconsciously been making choices surrounding food that may have landed you in the situation you're in right now. The 21-Day Hormone Makeover Meal Plan eliminates food groups that hijack hormones and contribute to weight gain, brain fog, and low energy, taking out the guesswork and leveraging science to reset your body to optimal functioning.

The Why Behind the Elimination

Sugar and sugar substitutes, gluten and other grains, eggs, caffeine, dairy, nightshades (optional), processed foods, and red meat take a hiatus from your diet for 21 days on this program. Why? These foods drive inflammation and may even be specifically causing some of your worst symptoms. I know that looking at that list is intimidating, but bear with me. These are very intentional choices to get rid of the most common culprits of hormone issues and menopausal symptoms that are linked to insulin resistance, estrogen dominance, thyroid dysfunction, and more. My recipes have already done the dirty work of removing these foods from your menu, so all you have to do is follow them!

Let's take a quick tour of the risks these foods expose your hormones to:

Sugar and sugar substitutes cause insulin spikes that lead to excess fat storage (especially around your belly) and also affect your cortisol levels, which in turn disrupt your delicate estrogen/progesterone balance.

Gluten creates an inflammatory response in your gut, brain, and thyroid.

Grains and corn increase gut inflammation, which contributes to digestive issues, leaky gut, and irritable bowel and decreases the number of essential substances (such as serotonin) that are produced in your intestines.

Caffeine revs up those adrenal stress hormones that send your body into survival mode day in and day out. If you've spent your adult life timing your day based on when you get your next shot of espresso, we are going to establish new patterns that won't sabotage your healing.

Dairy can cause inflammation in your body or exacerbate already existing issues, especially if your body doesn't digest lactose or casein well.

Nightshade intolerances lead to inflammation in certain people, causing digestive issues, acne, and joint pain. If you know that you have a sensitivity to nightshades, I recommend removing them from the program. If you think you may have a sensitivity, feel free to remove them for these 21 days and reintroduce them during the reentry phase.

Processed foods and meats are loaded with hormone impostors that you definitely do not need to be ingesting. These substances can create an estrogen-dominant state in your body that is responsible for the specific symptoms.

Red meat is probably the elimination choice I get the most pushback on. But hear me out: Consuming red meat regularly raises your estrogen levels. If you're in perimenopause or menopause, you likely already have too high a concentration of estrogen in your body in the first place, so this is an easy switch to prevent estrogen dominance from worsening. Red meat is also associated with consuming less fiber, which is necessary for eliminating the bad estrogens from your body. This puts an extra detoxifying burden on your liver and causes the growth of bad gut bacteria, which strains your digestive health.

Eating with Intent and Purpose

The intention of this 21-Day Hormone Makeover Program is not to make you feel deprived. It's to give you a chance to evaluate every area of your life and make mindful choices to heal your symptoms and get your body back on track. Nutrition is just one piece of the puzzle, but sticking to these guidelines is essential if you want to achieve your best results.

1. Stick to the Yes/No food lists. These are essential for creating and maintaining the success you are desperate for. Even giving in once to coffee, sugar, gluten, dairy, or the other foods on the No list can set your success back substantially. Give me these three weeks, then we'll talk about how to reintroduce these foods if you decide you want to.
2. Be mindful of portion control by using a smaller plate. Healthy food on small plates will train your eyes to see fullness before you experience it. Smaller plates make you think you're getting more, rather than using a large plate and feeling like you need to put more on it. Make sure each meal incorporates fibrous vegetables, healthy fat, and protein. This trio will keep you full longer between the three meals.
3. Incorporate smoothies or shakes into each day. This is the best, most efficient way to give your body what it needs to thrive when you use quality protein powder, fiber, and superfoods.

21-Day Hormone Makeover Yes/No Foods List

Yes Foods

Legumes

Black beans	Mung beans	Kidney beans
Garbanzo beans	White beans	Pinto and pink beans
Adzuki beans	Lima beans	Tempeh, organic non-GMO

Protein: Meats, Poultry, Fish, and Plant-Based

Organic whole chicken, chicken breast and thighs	Organic bone-in turkey breast or thighs, ground turkey	Wild salmon
		Black cod
		All whitefish
Organic and fermented tofu	Anchovies	Tuna
Organic and fermented tempeh	Wild shrimp and scallops	

Fruits

Apples	Berries (strawberries, blackberries, raspberries, blueberries)	Lemons
Avocados		Grapefruits
Cherries		Oranges
	Limes	Pomegranates
		Olives

Starchy Vegetables

Butternut squash	Plantains	Summer squash
Carrots	Pumpkin	Winter squash
Parsnips	Sweet potatoes	Yams

Non-Starchy Vegetables

Artichokes
Arugula
Asparagus
Beets
Bell peppers
Bok choy
Broccoli
Broccoli rabe (rapini)
Broccoli sprouts
Brussels sprouts
Cabbage
Cauliflower
Celery
Chard

Cucumbers
Dandelion greens
Eggplants
Endives
Fennel
Garlic
Gingerroot
Green onion
Green beans
Jalapeño
Kale/baby kale
Leeks
Lettuce (all types)
Microgreens

Mixed greens
Onions
Peas
Radishes
Serrano chiles
Shallots
Snow peas
Spinach
Tomatoes
Tatsoi
Watercress
Zucchini

Sea Vegetables

Nori
Kombu

Hijiki
Arame

Dulse

Seeds and Nuts

Raw pumpkin seeds
Raw sunflower seeds
Almonds

Cashews
Brazil nuts
Pine nuts

Pistachios
Walnuts

Herbal Teas

Chamomile
Matcha
Mint
Tulsi (holy basil)

Rooibos
Dandelion root
Green tea
Ginger

Lemon balm
Peppermint

Herbs and Spices

Whole black peppercorns

Whole bay leaf

Ground cardamom

Ground cumin and cumin seeds

Ground paprika

Ground chili powder

Ground coriander

Ground cinnamon and sticks

Ground curry powder

Turmeric

Ground/fresh ginger

Ground nutmeg

Dried/fresh basil

Dried/fresh cilantro (or coriander)

Dried/fresh oregano

Dried/fresh parsley

Dried/fresh rosemary

Dried/fresh sage

Dried/fresh thyme

Dried/fresh dill

Oils and Vinegars

Extra-virgin olive oil

Virgin coconut oil

Avocado oil

Raw apple cider vinegar

Raw organic coconut vinegar

Red wine vinegar

Other Ingredients

Broth: bone, chicken, vegetable

Brown mustard/ Dijon mustard

Coconut milk

Coconut aminos

High-quality sea salt

Tahini

Sauerkraut/ fermented vegetables/kimchi

Unsweetened almond milk

Maca powder

Cocoa nibs

No Foods

Grains

Wheat

Rye

Spelt

Kamut

Oats (cross-contaminated with gluten)

Buckwheat (cross-contaminated with gluten)

Millet (cross-contaminated with gluten)

Sorghum (cross-contaminated with gluten)

Lentils (cross-contaminated with gluten)

Rice

Quinoa

Dairy

Milk	Whey	Evaporated milk
Cream	Ice cream	Whipped cream
Yogurt	Sour cream	Sweetened condensed milk
Cheese	Cream cheese	
Butter/ghee	Cottage cheese	

Meat

Processed meat	Pork	Eggs
Processed beef	Lard	
Red meat	Tallow	

Soy

Soy milk	Textured vegetable protein	Tempeh (unless organic and fermented)
Soy oil	Tofu (unless organic and fermented)	Tamari and soy sauce
Soy protein isolate		Soy lecithin
Soy protein powder		

Corn

Corn on the cob	Masa	Baking powder
Frozen cob	Polenta	Dextrose
Corn tortillas	Cornmeal	Sorbitol
Hominy	Corn flour	Maltodextrin
Grits	Cornstarch	Food starch

| Vegetable starch | Vegetable protein | Xanthan gum |
| Vegetable gum | High fructose corn syrup | |

Nuts

Peanuts

Nightshades (Only if You Can't Tolerate Them)

Tomatoes	White potatoes	Mexican seasoning
Tomatillos	Goji berries	Taco seasoning
Peppers (sweet and hot)	Hot sauce	Chili powder
Eggplant	Cayenne pepper	Chipotle chili powder
	Curry powder	

Sugar

| Cane sugar | Agave nectar | Honey |
| Sucanat | Maple syrup | Sugar substitutes |

Other Foods

| Alcohol | Chocolate | Margarine |
| Caffeine | Refined vegetable oils | Butter substitutes |

21-Day Hormone Makeover Meal Plan

Cooking and eating hormone-loving foods shouldn't add to your stress. Use the 21-Day Meal Plan I've provided with day-by-day suggestions as a framework, and have fun finding what works with your lifestyle and your body.

Guidelines

- This meal plan is not super rigid or set in stone. As long as you're using the Yes list ingredients and recipes provided as guidelines, you have a lot of flexibility!
- Use any of the recipes as a substitute for any of the ones included on the daily meal plans.
- If you have leftovers, use them for lunch or dinner the next day.
- If you're out of one ingredient, sub it for something else on your approved shopping list.
- Anti-inflammatory smoothies and shakes in the morning fuel your body with protein, fiber, and superfoods. Feel free to sub a smoothie or shake in for lunch or dinner if you are on the go.

Meal Plan for 21 Days

Day 1

Breakfast
Lemon Ginger Gut-Restoring Tea (page 306)
Strawberry Chocolate Bliss Shake (page 311)

Lunch
Build Your Own Salad (pick one or create your own) (page 318)
1 small apple, or 1/2 cup berries

Dinner
Salmon Fillets with Lemon and Garlic (page 325)
Steamed spinach with lemon

Day 2

Breakfast
Lemon Ginger Gut-Restoring Tea or tulsi tea (page 306)
Dr. Mariza's Chocolate Cake Shake (page 312)

Lunch

Mexican Chopped Salad or leftover salmon fillets with mixed greens
  (page 322)

½ sliced apple and 1 tablespoon unsweetened almond butter

2 tablespoons sauerkraut or fermented vegetables (optional)

Dinner

Build Your Own Bowl (pick one or create your own) (page 314)

Mixed green salad with vinaigrette or Build Your Own Salad (page 318)

Day 3

Breakfast

Golden milk, herbal, or tulsi tea

Hormone-Loving Bone Broth (optional) (page 332)

Dr. Mariza's Hormone Love Smoothie (page 310)

Lunch

Healthy Curry Chicken Salad on Mixed Greens (page 323)

½ cup sliced strawberries

2 tablespoons sauerkraut or fermented vegetables (optional)

Dinner

Turkey Meatballs with Spaghetti Squash and Cherry Tomato–Basil
  Sauce (page 327)

Mixed green salad with vinaigrette or Build Your Own Salad (page 318)

Day 4

Breakfast

Lemon Ginger Gut-Restoring Tea (page 306)

Strawberry Chocolate Bliss Shake (page 311)

Lunch

Healthy Curry Chicken Salad leftovers or Build Your Own Salad (pick
  one or create your own) (page 323 or page 318)

½ sliced apple and 1 tablespoon unsweetened almond butter

Dinner

Sautéed Shrimp with Lemon and Parsley with Spaghetti Squash and
Creamy Zesty Pesto (page 326 and page 341)

Day 5

Breakfast

Tulsi or green tea

Hormone-Loving Bone Broth (optional) (page 332)

Blueberry Matcha Smoothie (page 313)

Lunch

Healthy Italian Tuna Salad (page 326)

$1/2$ cup mixed berries

2 tablespoons sauerkraut or fermented vegetables (optional)

Dinner

Chicken Fajitas with Cauliflower Rice (page 329)

Mixed green salad with vinaigrette or Build Your Own Salad (page 318)

Dr. Mariza's Guacamole (page 340)

Day 6

Breakfast

Lemon Ginger Gut-Restoring Tea or tulsi tea (page 306)

Dr. Mariza's Chocolate Cake Shake (page 312)

Lunch

Healthy Italian Tuna Salad leftovers or Build Your Own Salad
(pick one or create your own) (page 326 or page 318)

Dinner

Creamy Chicken and Veggie Soup (page 333)

Build Your Own Salad (pick one or create your own) (page 318)

Day 7

Breakfast
Green or herbal tea
Ultimate Anti-inflammatory Green Smoothie (page 312)

Lunch
Creamy Chicken and Veggie Soup leftovers (page 333)
Build Your Own Salad (pick one or create your own) (page 318)

Dinner
Grilled Halibut with Strawberry-Avocado Salsa (page 324)
Cauliflower Rice (page 339)
Mixed green salad with vinaigrette or Build Your Own Salad (page 318)

Day 8

Breakfast
Golden milk, herbal, or tulsi tea
Hormone-Loving Bone Broth (optional) (page 332)
Dr. Mariza's Hormone Love Smoothie (page 310)

Lunch
Build Your Own Bowl (pick one or create your own) (page 314)
2 tablespoons sauerkraut or fermented vegetables (optional)

Dinner
Easy Turkey Burger (page 331)
Baked Sweet Potato Fries (page 341)

Day 9

Breakfast
Lemon Ginger Gut-Restoring Tea (page 306)
Strawberry Chocolate Bliss Shake (page 311)

Lunch

Easy Turkey Burger leftovers or Build Your Own Salad (pick one or create your own) (page 331 or page 318)

Dinner

Salmon Fillets with Lemon and Garlic (page 325)

Brussels sprouts with garlic and pine nuts

Day 10

Breakfast

Lemon Ginger Gut-Restoring Tea or tulsi tea (page 306)

Dr. Mariza's Chocolate Cake Shake (page 312)

Lunch

Mexican Chopped Salad with protein of choice (page 322)

$1/2$ cup of mixed berries

2 tablespoons sauerkraut or fermented vegetables (optional)

Dinner

Creamy Sweet Potato and Carrot Soup (page 335)

Mixed green salad with vinaigrette with protein of choice

Day 11

Breakfast

Golden milk, herbal, or tulsi tea

Hormone-Loving Bone Broth (optional) (page 332)

Dr. Mariza's Hormone Love Smoothie (page 310)

Lunch

Creamy Sweet Potato and Carrot Soup leftovers or Build Your Own Salad (pick one or create your own) (page 335 or page 318)

Dinner

Turkey Meatballs with Spaghetti Squash and Creamy Zesty Pesto (page 327)

Mixed green salad with vinaigrette or Build Your Own Salad (page 318)

Day 12

Breakfast
Green or herbal tea
Ultimate Anti-inflammatory Green Smoothie (page 312)

Lunch
Turkey Meatballs with Spaghetti Squash and Creamy Zesty Pesto
leftovers or Build Your Own Salad (pick one or create your own)
(page 327 or page 318)

Dinner
Healthy Curry Chicken Salad on Mixed Greens (page 323)
Baked Sweet Potato Fries (page 341)

Day 13

Breakfast
Golden milk, herbal, or tulsi tea
Strawberry Chocolate Bliss Shake (page 311)

Lunch
Healthy Curry Chicken Salad leftovers or Build Your Own Bowl (pick
one or create your own) (page 323 or page 314)

Dinner
Sautéed Shrimp with Lemon and Parsley (page 326)
Cauliflower Rice (page 339)
Sautéed Garlic Vegetables (page 340)

Day 14

Breakfast
Lemon Ginger Gut-Restoring Tea or tulsi tea (page 306)
Dr. Mariza's Chocolate Cake Shake (page 312)

Lunch

Build Your Own Bowl (pick one or create your own) with leftover
Cauliflower Rice (page 314 or page 339)

1/2 cup mixed berries

2 tablespoons sauerkraut or fermented vegetables (optional)

Dinner

Chard and White Bean Soup (page 332)

Build Your Own Salad (pick one or create your own) (page 318)

Day 15

Breakfast

Tulsi or green tea

Hormone-Loving Bone Broth (optional) (page 332)

Blueberry Matcha Smoothie (page 313)

Lunch

Chard and White Bean Soup leftovers or Build Your Own Bowl (pick
one or create your own) (page 332 or page 314)

Dinner

Easy Turkey Burger (page 331)

Baked Sweet Potato Fries (page 341)

Dr. Mariza's Guacamole (page 340)

Day 16

Breakfast

Lemon Ginger Gut-Restoring Tea or herbal tea (page 306)

Strawberry Chocolate Bliss Shake (page 311)

Lunch

Healthy Italian Tuna Salad (page 326)

1/2 cup mixed berries

2 tablespoons sauerkraut or fermented vegetables (optional)

Dinner
Build Your Own Bowl (pick one or create your own) (page 314)
Mixed green salad

Day 17

Breakfast
Green or herbal tea
Hormone-Loving Bone Broth (optional) (page 332)
Ultimate Anti-inflammatory Green Smoothie (page 312)

Lunch
Healthy Italian Tuna Salad leftovers or Build Your Own Salad (pick
   one or create your own) (page 326 or page 318)

Dinner
Creamy Chicken and Veggie Soup (page 333)
Build Your Own Salad (pick one or create your own) (page 318)

Day 18

Breakfast
Golden milk, herbal, or tulsi tea
Dr. Mariza's Hormone Love Smoothie (page 310)

Lunch
Healthy Curry Chicken Salad on Mixed Greens (page 323)
$1/2$ cup mixed berries

Dinner
Grilled Halibut with Strawberry-Avocado Salsa (page 324)
Cauliflower Rice (page 339)

Day 19

Breakfast

Lemon Ginger Gut-Restoring Tea or tulsi tea (page 306)

Dr. Mariza's Chocolate Cake Shake (page 312)

Lunch

Healthy Curry Chicken Salad leftovers or Build Your Own Salad (pick one or create your own) (page 323 or page 318)

Dinner

Chicken Fajitas with Cauliflower Rice (page 329)

Dr. Mariza's Guacamole (page 340)

Day 20

Breakfast

Golden milk, herbal, or tulsi tea

Hormone-Loving Bone Broth (optional) (page 332)

Dr. Mariza's Hormone Love Smoothie (page 310)

Lunch

Chicken Fajitas leftovers with Build Your Own Salad (pick one or create your own) (page or page 318)

Dinner

Salmon Fillets with Lemon and Garlic (page 325)

Sautéed Garlic Vegetables (page 340)

Spaghetti Squash with Creamy Zesty Pesto (page 341)

Day 21

Breakfast

Green or herbal tea

Ultimate Anti-inflammatory Green Smoothie (page 312)

Lunch

Mexican Chopped Salad with protein of your choice (page 322)

Dinner

Turkey Meatballs with Spaghetti Squash and Cherry Tomato–Basil
Sauce (page 327)

21-Day Hormone Makeover Recipes

These recipes are designed to provide you with easy-to-create
smoothies for breakfast and simple, nutrient-dense meals for both
lunch and dinner. Many of the recipes were created by me and my
good friend and therapeutic chef, Anna V. Zulaica. She is also the co-
author of *The Dash Diet Cookbook, The Matcha Miracle,* and *The Low
G.I. Slow Cooker.* The recipes have been tested by me and many women
who have successfully completed the 21-Day Hormone Makeover
Program. These recipes really work to help your body heal and will
give you a framework for cooking healthy whole food meals without
complicated ingredients or cooking techniques. Creating a cooking-
at-home lifestyle is the key to sustainable hormonal balance, and the
principles you'll learn by following these recipes will set you up for
long-term success.

Beverages and Teas

I personally love delicious, healthy tonics, water infusions, lattes, and
teas to drink throughout the day. You will find recipes to add extra
flavor and sparkle to your water, while boosting your immunity and
taste buds. You will also find tonics and teas that focus on loving your
liver, gut, and adrenals. My favorite way to start my day is with a
Lemon Ginger Gut-Restoring tea. I also share my favorite matcha and
golden milk latte recipes to start your morning, or afternoon, off right.

Lemon-Lime Ginger Immunity Water

Boost your immunity and support your digestive system with this easy-to-make water infusion, combining lemon, lime, and ginger.

SERVES: 4

2 lemons, sliced into wheels

1 lime, sliced into wheels

3 inches fresh ginger, peeled and sliced

1 ½ quarts still, filtered water

Ice

Layer lemons, lime, and ginger slices along the bottom of a 2-quart pitcher. Cover with ice (to your liking) and top off with water. Allow to steep for at least 30 minutes, but preferably for 2–3 hours, before serving.

For an added detoxification boost, squeeze a full lemon into the water infusion after adding the lemon, lime, and ginger slices.

Strawberry Lemon Basil Spritzer

This is the perfect way to create healthy sparkling water. I use this recipe for picnics and parties.

SERVES: 4

2 cups strawberries, hulled and quartered

1 lemon, sliced into wheels

2–4 sprigs of basil, stems included

½ quart still water

1 quart sparkling water

Ice

In a 2-quart pitcher, arrange the fruit and basil at the bottom and cover with ice. Then pour water in to cover the ingredients. Allow the mixture to steep for at least 30 minutes, then top with sparkling water just before serving.

Like more or less fizz? Adjust amounts of still versus sparkling water accordingly! Just make sure the still water, sparkling water, and ingredients amounts to 2 quarts.

Liver Love Tonic

This anti-inflammatory liver tonic packs a punch. Dandelion greens, ginger, lemon, parsley, mint, and cinnamon are powerful for combating inflammation and giving the liver key antioxidants and nutrients to thrive.

SERVES: 2

4 cups filtered water

½ cup dandelion greens or mixed greens

2-inch piece of fresh ginger, peeled and sliced

Juice of 1 lemon

3–4 sprigs fresh parsley

8–10 fresh mint leaves

⅛ teaspoon cinnamon

Combine water, dandelion greens, ginger, lemon juice, parsley, mint, and cinnamon in the blender and blend until smooth, approximately 1 minute. Pour mixture into 2 small glasses and enjoy.

Adrenal Love Tulsi Tea

Tulsi, or holy basil, is an adaptogenic herb known to support adrenal function and lower stress levels. This tea is the perfect swap for caffeinated teas.

SERVES: 2

2 cups filtered water

2 tablespoons dried organic tulsi or 2 tulsi tea bags

2 teaspoons lemon juice

Boil filtered water and pour it over dried tulsi leaves using a tea strainer. Add lemon juice and stir. Pour tea into a cup and enjoy hot or warm.

Lemon Ginger Gut-Restoring Tea

This is the perfect tea to begin your morning. Lemon and ginger prime your digestive tract in the morning and offer immune boosting benefits.

SERVES: 1

2 cups filtered water

1 teaspoon freshly grated
   organic ginger

Juice of ½ lemon

Boil water in a teakettle or in a pot on the stove. Add fresh ginger and lemon juice to a tea infuser placed over your mug. Pour boiling water over the infuser into the cup and let the lemon and ginger steep for 5 minutes before enjoying.

Vanilla Turmeric Golden Milk Latte

Love your liver and cells with the benefits of turmeric in this rich and creamy golden milk latte. Curcumin, found in turmeric, boosts antioxidant levels, supports immune system function, and increases brain function.

SERVES: 1

1 cup organic coconut milk

1 cup organic unsweetened
   vanilla almond milk

1 tablespoon coconut oil or
   MCT oil

¼ teaspoon ground cinnamon

I drop Turmeric essential oil (or 1½ tsp ground turmeric)

¼ teaspoon ground ginger

I pinch ground black pepper

3–5 drops stevia, to taste (optional)

In a small saucepan, heat coconut milk and vanilla almond milk on low for 3–4 minutes. Whisk in coconut oil, Turmeric essential oil, ginger, black pepper, and stevia. Whisk to combine and warm over medium heat. Heat until hot to the touch but not boiling—about 4 minutes—whisking frequently. Remove from heat and pour into a mug, serving while hot to boost antioxidants and support your thyroid.

Iced Matcha Latte

My favorite green tea packs a massive antioxidant punch. Matcha boosts energy levels and supports a healthy metabolism. Matcha also contains L-theanine, designed to enhance cognitive function, memory, and focus.

MAKES 2 (8-OUNCE) SERVINGS

I teaspoon matcha green tea powder

14 ounces unsweetened vanilla almond milk or unsweetened coconut milk

Pinch of cinnamon (optional)

2–3 drops stevia (optional)

Place all ingredients in a blender. Blend on high for about 30 seconds until completely blended and a little frothy. Add a pinch of cinnamon, taste and adjust sweetener, if desired.

Serve over ice and enjoy!

Breakfast Smoothies and Shakes

Ready in as little as five minutes, protein shakes and green smoothies are the easiest and yummiest way to upgrade your health to look and feel your very best—fast! They are also easily digestible for optimal energy and focus, and they make a great postworkout recovery drink to boost fat burning and muscle repair.

Whether you call it a smoothie or shake, the key to a healthy meal replacement drink is a trifecta of **clean, lean protein, healthy fat**, and **plenty of fiber**. Add the right liquids with a healthy dose of greens, and you're all set with a complete, satisfying meal!

And guess what the perfect hormone-support trio is? That's right. Proteins, healthy fats, and fiber! Below you will find my top tips to help you create the ideal meal-on-the-go.

HOW TO MAKE A SMOOTHIE

Here are my top 5 tips for smoothie success:

1. **Be sure that you have a high-powered blender** to get a smoothie and not a chunky! Vitamix, Blendtec, or NutriBullet blenders work the best for the creamiest version.
2. **Use a liquid base and a sufficient blend time.** This is the secret to a smooth, creamy green smoothie! Put your liquid in first, filling it up to the 2.5- to 3-cup mark for 2 quarts of smoothie. Since we avoid dairy, I like to use coconut water or water as a base, or for a creamier version, swap in unsweetened almond milk or coconut milk.
3. **Pile in 2–4 cups of packed, freshly washed greens.** Combine leafy greens and green plants like kale, spinach, lettuce, parsley, mint, or whatever you like. Greens are the most nutrient-dense food available, so pack it in! If you are a newbie, start with spinach for a milder flavor.
4. **Now blend it up!** I recommend at least 45 seconds; otherwise, you will end up with chunks of greens.

5. **Add in about 1 cup of your favorite frozen fruits.** Go for low-sugar options like berries, but whatever is in season usually makes a great choice. Blend up your smoothie one more time and you're all set!

HOW TO MAKE YOUR SMOOTHIE A COMPLETE MEAL

To take your green smoothie to the next level and make it a complete meal, here are 3 things you can add to make sure you are satisfied and full for 4 to 6 hours. This way, you'll be able to ward off snacking and cravings that could derail your success!

I. ADD IN YOUR ESSENTIALLY WHOLE® PURE DAILY FIBER.

Did you know that the average American woman consumes less than 12 grams of fiber each day, but **we need between 35 to 45 grams every day**? Adding daily fiber to your smoothies will give you the daily dose needed to heal your gut and support your hormones.

It's the key so many of you may be missing to keeping your bowel movements regular and your estrogen in balance!

2. ADD A HORMONE-FRIENDLY DAILY PROTEIN POWDER (PALEO OR PEA AS A VEGAN OPTION).

As you get older, the key to feeling your best is to maintain your muscle mass, particularly if you're someone like me who has lost weight or wants to lose weight. Maintaining muscle mass is associated with greater longevity.

3. ADD HEALTHY FAT.

Fats are the building blocks of hormones, so making sure you have enough healthy fat daily is critical for keeping your body in balance. They will also help you feel full longer to help ward off cravings between meals.

My favorite way to add a luscious, creamy texture and a dose of healthy fat is by adding **avocado** to my smoothies. Packed with heart- and hormone-loving monounsaturated fats, avocados are the secret ingredient to take your smoothie to the next level!

Another alternative is to add a tablespoon or two of **coconut butter** (or **coconut oil**, if that's what you have on hand).

Now that you have everything you need to make your smoothie a complete meal, here are some of my favorite recipes you can begin incorporating into your daily routine.

Dr. Mariza's Hormone Love Smoothie

Get ready to love your hormones with this nutrient-packed smoothie. In just 5 minutes you have everything you need to balance your hormones in one smoothie. Healthy fats, clean protein powder, and fiber are the cornerstone ingredients to support your liver and gut. Maca is great for estrogen metabolism, and energy and berries add the perfect amount of sweetness and antioxidants.

SERVES: 1

2 cups baby kale or spinach

½ cup purified water

1 cup unsweetened vanilla almond milk or coconut milk

Juice of ½ lemon

½ medium avocado, pitted, peeled, and chopped

1 cup frozen raspberries and/ or blueberries

1–2 scoops Essentially Whole® Vanilla Protein (or similar protein powder)

2 teaspoons Essentially Whole® Pure Daily Fiber (or 1 tablespoon freshly ground flaxseed)

½ tablespoon maca powder (optional)

Add the kale or spinach, water, and unsweetened vanilla almond milk to a high-powered blender. Start blending on low and, as the kale starts to break down, increase to medium speed until completely broken down and smooth. Add lemon juice, avocado, frozen berries, vanilla protein powder, fiber, and maca (if desired). Blend well on medium to high speed until desired consistency is achieved, about 1 minute. Enjoy immediately!

Strawberry Chocolate Bliss Shake

SERVES: 1

2 cups mixed greens

1 cup purified water

1 cup unsweetened coconut milk

1 cup frozen strawberries

2 teaspoons Essentially Whole® Daily Fiber (or 1 tablespoon freshly ground flaxseed)

1 tablespoon almond or cashew butter

1-2 scoops Essentially Whole® Paleo Daily Protein Chocolate (or similar protein powder)

2 teaspoons unsweetened baking cocoa (optional)

Add the greens, water, and unsweetened coconut milk to a high-powered blender. Start blending on low, and increase to medium speed until greens are completely broken down and smooth. Add the frozen strawberries, fiber, almond butter, chocolate protein powder, and unsweetened baking cocoa (if desired). Blend well on medium to high speed until desired consistency is achieved, about 1 minute. Enjoy immediately!

Ultimate Anti-inflammatory Green Smoothie

Your liver and brain will love you for drinking this smoothie in the morning! Turmeric, cinnamon, matcha, and coconut oil boost cognitive function and alertness. Berries, turmeric, and matcha are powerful antioxidants for liver detoxification. Drink this smoothie knowing your body will love you for it!

SERVES: 1

2½ cups greens

1 ½ cups coconut water

½ cup unsweetened coconut milk

½ cup frozen blueberries

¼ cup frozen raspberries

2 teaspoons Essentially Whole® Daily Fiber (or 1 tablespoon freshly ground flaxseed)

1 tablespoon coconut oil or MCT oil

¼ teaspoon cinnamon

½ teaspoon turmeric

1–2 scoops Essentially Whole® Vanilla Protein (or similar protein powder)

1 teaspoon matcha

Add the greens, water, and unsweetened coconut milk to a high-powered blender. Start blending on low and increase to medium speed until greens are completely broken down and smooth. Add frozen berries, fiber, coconut oil, cinnamon, turmeric, vanilla protein powder, and matcha. Blend well on medium to high speed until desired consistency is achieved, about 1 minute. Enjoy immediately!

Dr. Mariza's Chocolate Cake Shake

I created this smoothie out of a desire to make a delicious chocolate shake that included healthy fats, clean protein, and liver-loving antioxidants. Maca is ideal for energy, estrogen metabolism, and mood. Cacao nibs are a great source of antioxidants, magnesium, fiber, and flavonoids to support healthy brain and heart function. This dessert smoothie packs a hormone-loving punch.

SERVES: 1

2 cups spinach or mixed greens

1 tablespoon almond or cashew butter

⅛ teaspoon real vanilla extract

1 tablespoon cacao nibs

½ medium avocado, chopped

1–2 scoops Essentially Whole® Chocolate Protein (or similar protein powder)

2 teaspoons Essentially Whole® Daily Fiber (or 1 tablespoon freshly ground flaxseed)

2 cups unsweetened vanilla almond milk or coconut milk

½ tablespoon maca powder (optional)

½ cup ice

Add the greens and unsweetened almond milk to a blender. Start blending on low and as greens start to break down, increase to medium speed until greens are completely broken down and smooth. Add almond butter, vanilla extract, cacao nibs, avocado, protein powder, fiber, almond milk, maca powder (if desired), and ice and blend well on medium to high speed until desired consistency is achieved, about 1 minute. Serve immediately.

Tip: *Sprinkle cacao nibs on top of your smoothie for added crunch and polyphenol antioxidants.*

Blueberry Matcha Smoothie

SERVES: 2

2 cups mixed greens

2 cups water

Juice of ½ lime

1 small avocado, pitted, peeled and chopped

1 cup frozen blueberries

I teaspoon matcha green tea

1-2 scoops Essentially
  Whole® Vanilla Protein
  (or similar protein
  powder)

2 teaspoons Essentially
  Whole® Daily Fiber (or
  I tablespoon freshly
  ground flaxseed)

3-4 ice cubes (optional)

Add the mixed greens and water to a high-powered blender. Start blending on low and, as greens start to break down, increase to medium speed until completely broken down and smooth, approximately 45-60 seconds. Add lime juice, avocado, blueberries, matcha, vanilla protein powder, fiber, and ice. Blend well on medium to high speed until desired consistency is achieved, about I minute. Enjoy immediately.

Lunch and Dinner Entrees

Build Your Own Bowl Guide

Bowls are a quick, easy-to-put-together option and most can be enjoyed cold or hot. Mix and match your starches, proteins, vegetables, and toppings. It's a great option for family meals because picky eaters can build their own bowls and mix and match ingredients to their liking. By batch cooking the ingredients, you can try different-style bowls or salads for several days in a row and just switch up the toppings and sauce/dressing. I think of building the perfect bowl of food as working in layers.

General Ratio for I bowl for I person

Layer I—Base: I cup

Layer 2—Vegetables: 2 cups

Layer 3—Protein: 3-4 ounces (general rule of thumb: size of your palm)

Layer 4—Superfoods: 1-2 tablespoons (depending on potency of flavor), $1/2$ avocado

Layer 5—Dressing/Sauce: 2-3 tablespoons

Layer 1: Base (1 cup)

- Any items from the Legumes list (example: black beans, white beans)
- Any items from the Starchy Vegetables list (example: butternut squash, plantains, sweet potatoes)
- Any item from the Non-Starchy Vegetables list (example: cauliflower rice, sautéed spinach)
- Ideas for creating the base: Use a spiralizer to make zoodles, or noodles from butternut squash or sweet potatoes.
- Beans: Presoaking beans before cooking helps cut down cooking time and reduces bloat and gas once cooked. Canned beans are okay to use, but make sure to rinse before consuming, as some have added salt.

Layer 2: Veggies (2 cups)

- Any items from the Non-Starchy Vegetables list
- Pickled veggies ($1/4$ cup)

Layer 3: Protein (3 to 4 ounces, or the size of the palm of your hand)

- Any item from the Meats, Poultry, and Fish list
- If you do not eat meat, make sure to include legumes for your protein

Layer 4: Superfoods

Consider these your toppings.

- Healthy fats: 1 to 2 tablespoons seeds, 2 tablespoons chopped nuts, $1/2$ avocado
- Fermented veggies: $1/4$ cup kimchi, 2 tablespoons sauerkraut
- Chopped herbs: 1 tablespoon

Layer 5: Dressing/Sauce 1-2 tablespoons

- Olive oil
- Avocado oil
- Apple cider vinegar
- Red wine vinegar
- Lemon juice
- Homemade dressing
- Avocado sauce
- Salsa/pico de gallo
- Pesto

Build Your Own Bowl Inspirations

Baja Bowl

Layer 1: Cauliflower rice
Layer 2: Black beans, sautéed spinach and mushrooms
Layer 3: Pan-fried or roasted skinless, boneless chicken thigh
Layer 4: Chopped cilantro, chopped jalapeño peppers (the avocado in the dressing below counts as a healthy fat)
Layer 5: Avocado Sauce (see recipe below)

Avocado Sauce

SERVES: 4

1 medium avocado, pitted

¼ cup cilantro, chopped

Juice of 1 lime

½ medium white onion, chopped

¼ teaspoon garlic powder

½ teaspoon sea salt

½ teaspoon cracked black pepper

Optional: ½ jalapeño or serrano chile, chopped finely

¼ cup filtered water

Add all ingredients to a blender or food processor with ¼ cup water and blend until smooth. If it's too thick, add more water, 1 tablespoon at a time. Serve on top of Baja Bowl, or any other bowl or recipe if you love avocado like me.

Mediterranean Bowl

Layer 1: Roasted butternut squash
Layer 2: Roasted zucchini, cauliflower, steamed or sautéed kale, stems removed and cut into thin ribbons
Layer 3: Pan-fried or roasted salmon fillet
Layer 4: Chopped fresh basil, chili flakes, toasted pine nuts
Layer 5: Low-sodium premade or homemade pesto (see recipe on page 329)

Thai Coconut Curry Bowl

Layer 1: Zoodles (spiralize zucchini, broccoli stems, or sweet potato for this base)
Layer 2: Bell pepper, onion, green beans
Layer 3: Diced-chicken breast
Layer 4: Pumpkin seeds, Thai basil, cilantro
Layer 5: Curried coconut milk sauce

For curried coconut milk sauce, sauté premade Thai curry paste (no MSG and no soy) in a large pot with coconut oil. Add diced bell pepper, onion, and green beans and sauté for about three minutes. Add chicken breast and a splash of water to the deglaze pot. Sauté for about two minutes, then add two 16-ounce cans coconut milk along with Thai basil and cilantro. Simmer for about 10 minutes to let flavors infuse.

Zoodles (from zucchini) and broccoli noodles can be sautéed in a pan, lightly steamed, or enjoyed raw. Sweet potato zoodles are not recommended to be eaten raw.

Buddha Bowl

Layer 1: Mung beans or beans of choice and steamed or
roasted sweet potato

Layer 2: Steamed broccoli, bok choy, or any vegetable from
the Non-Starchy Vegetables list, seaweed

Layer 3: Steamed, roasted, or pan-fried black cod, or salmon

Layer 4: Avocado, nori flakes or furikake, kimchi, chopped
green onion

Layer 5: Tahini dressing (recipe on page 339), dash of coconut
aminos

This is a very flexible dish. It can be enjoyed cold or hot. Mix and
match your proteins and vegetables.

Build Your Own Salad Guide

Salads are an easy way to create an easy nutrient-dense lunch or dinner with all colors of the rainbow. Every Sunday I prep my salad ingredients for the week by chopping and slicing vegetables and berries
and then organizing everything in glass Pyrex containers. This makes
it very easy to make a salad in five minutes. I also love to batch my vinaigrette dressings. One great tip is to make a large batch of dressing to
keep on hand at all times. Store in a mason jar, use painter's tape and
label and date the front of the jar so you can keep track of what it is
and how old it is. Oil-based vinaigrettes can last more than a month
in your refrigerator! If your oil seizes up or separates, let the jar sit at
room temperature or set it by your warm stove to liquefy it again. Give
it a shake and enjoy!

General Ratio for 1 salad for 1 person

Layer 1—Greens: 3–4 cups

Layer 2—Starch: 1 1/2 cups

Layer 3—Protein: 3–4 ounces (general rule of thumb is the size of your palm)

Layer 4—Vegetables/Fruit: 1–2 cups

Layer 5—Superfoods: 1–2 tablespoons (depending on potency of flavor), 1/2 avocado

Layer 6—Dressing: 1–2 tablespoons

Layer 1: Greens (3–4 cups)

- Arugula
- Spinach
- Kale
- Spring mix
- Power green mix (store-bought mix)
- Watercress (pretty powerful flavor, so you can mix with other greens)
- Tatsoi
- Nasturtium
- Dandelion greens
- Butter lettuce
- Romaine lettuce
- Any item from the Non-Starchy Vegetables list

Layer 2: Starch (1 1/2 cups)

Any item from the Legumes and/or Starchy Vegetables list

Layer 3: Protein (3–4 ounces)

- Any item from the Meats, Poultry, and Fish list
- If you do not eat meat, make sure to include legumes for your protein

Layer 4: Veggies/Fruits (1-2 cups)

- Any items from the Non-Starchy Vegetables list
- Any item from the Fruits list
- Pickled/fermented veggies (pickled onion, pickled radish, sauerkraut, kimchi)

Layer 5: Superfoods (1-2 tablespoons)

Consider these your toppings.
- Healthy fats: 1 to 2 tablespoons seeds, 2 tablespoons chopped nuts, $1/2$ avocado
- Fermented veggies: $1/4$ cup kimchi, 2 tablespoons sauerkraut
- Chopped herbs: 1-2 tablespoons

Layer 6: Dressing/Sauce (1-2 tablespoons)

- Any recipe from the homemade vinaigrettes, Tahini
- Dressing, or Creamy Green Goddess Dressing (recipes in Dressings section, page 337)

Build Your Own Salad Inspirations

Veggie-Inspired Niçoise Salad

Layer 1: Romaine or butter lettuce, chopped
Layer 2: Roasted or steamed sweet potatoes, large cubes
Layer 3: Canned albacore tuna in water
Layer 4: Steamed green beans, cut into 2-inch pieces, cherry tomatoes, halved, olives, radishes (thinly sliced or quartered)
Layer 5: Avocado, chopped walnuts
Layer 6: Red wine vinaigrette with chopped thyme and parsley

Warm Kale Salad

Layer 1: Kale—Destemmed, cut into $1/2$-inch ribbons and washed well, sautéed in olive oil or coconut oil

Layer 2: Roasted small diced sweet potato or butternut squash

Layer 3: Roasted turkey breast, thinly sliced, or any item from the Meats, Poultry, and Fish list

Layer 4: Small peeled diced apple tossed in a little lemon juice before adding to dish so they don't oxidize/brown

Layer 5: Toasted pine nuts

Layer 6: Simple Lemon Vinaigrette (page 336)

The Green Goddess Salad

Layer 1: Mixed greens

Layer 2: Garbanzo beans

Layer 3: Roasted chicken breast or organic, non-GMO tempeh, cubed

Layer 4: Blueberries, shredded carrot, alfalfa sprouts, pickled red onion

Layer 5: Toasted chopped pistachios

Layer 6: Creamy Green Goddess Dressing (page 338) or dressing of your choice

Pickled Red Onion

SERVES: 10–12

1 red onion, sliced paper thin

1 cup red wine vinegar

1 bay leaf

¼ teaspoon black peppercorns

Salt, to taste

Cut a red onion lengthwise/vertically so the root ball is still attached on both sides. Cut each half again horizontally and peel off the outer layer of skin. Use a mandoline slicer or a chef knife to slice paper-thin slices from one quarter of the onion.

In a small saucepan, heat red wine vinegar with bay leaf, black peppercorns, and a pinch of salt. Heat until salt dissolves. Add onions to a 16-ounce mason jar and pour the hot vinegar over them. Push them down until they are fully submerged. Let sit until they soften, about 20 minutes. Place the jar in the refrigerator to cool and store for up to a month. Add to salads and main dishes for extra flavor.

Autumn-Inspired Salad

Layer 1: Arugula

Layer 2: Roasted winter squash of choice, small dice (butternut squash, acorn squash, curry squash, kabocha squash, etc.), roasted or boiled peeled beets, cut into 1/2-inch cubes

Layer 3: Any item from the Meats, Poultry, and Fish list

Layer 4: Raw, thinly shaved fennel bulb

Layer 5: Pomegranate seeds, pumpkin seeds

Layer 6: Herbal Vinaigrette Dressing (page 337)

Mexican Chopped Salad

SERVES: 4

2 cups romaine lettuce, chopped

1 cup kale, chopped

1 cup purple cabbage, chopped

1 can (15.5 ounces) black beans, rinsed and drained

5 Roma tomatoes, cubed

1 ½ cups cucumber, chopped with skin on

½ medium avocado, pitted, peeled, and chopped

¼ cup white onion, diced, or very thinly sliced

¼ cup lime juice

⅛ cup extra virgin olive oil

2 tablespoons fresh cilantro, chopped

Salt and pepper to taste

In a large bowl, combine the romaine, kale, purple cabbage, black beans, tomatoes, cucumber, avocado, and onion. Pour the lime juice and olive oil over the salad and toss well. Season with cilantro and salt and pepper and serve along with a protein of your choice.

Tip: *Add grilled fish, or any protein, to this salad to make it a complete meal.*

Healthy Curry Chicken Salad on Mixed Greens

SERVES: 4

2 large boneless, skinless chicken breasts

½ cup carrots, chopped

1 cup beets, cooked and shredded

2 celery stalks, diced

1 medium avocado, pitted and diced

¼ cup fresh cilantro and/or parsley, chopped

1 tablespoon tahini (optional)

½ tablespoon red wine vinegar

1 teaspoon curry powder

⅛ teaspoon cinnamon

4 cups mixed greens

8 cherry tomatoes, sliced

¼ cup cashews

Trim the fat off the chicken and cut the breasts into fourths. Fill a medium pot with water and bring to a boil. Add the chicken and boil for 8–10 minutes, or until the centers are no longer pink. Strain the chicken and set it aside to cool.

In a separate bowl, combine the carrots, beets, and celery. Shred the cooled chicken with two forks and add to the bowl. Add the avocado, fresh cilantro and/or parsley, tahini (if desired), vinegar, curry powder, and cinnamon and mix well. Refrigerate for 30 minutes.

On top of the mixed greens add the chicken salad, top with the cherry tomatoes and cashews and serve.

Note: *Feel free to sub out chicken for tofu as a plant-based protein source.*

Main Dishes

Grilled Halibut with Strawberry-Avocado Salsa

SERVES: 4

I ripe medium avocado, pitted and cut into ½-inch chunks

8 ounces strawberries, hulled and cut into ¾-inch cubes

I cup cherry tomatoes, quartered

I jalapeño, seeded and minced

I tablespoon fresh cilantro, minced

2 tablespoons lime juice, divided

4 halibut or mahi-mahi fillets (4 to 6 ounces each), skin on

2 tablespoons extra-virgin olive oil

½ teaspoon coarse sea salt, divided

¼ teaspoon ground black pepper

I lime, cut into 4 wedges

Pinch of salt

Prepare a grill to medium-high heat.

Gently combine the avocado, strawberries, tomatoes, jalapeño, cilantro, and I tablespoon lime juice in a large mixing bowl. Season salsa to taste with salt and pepper and set aside at room temperature.

Place fish fillets in a 13 x 9 x 2-inch glass baking dish. Brush with the olive oil and remaining lime juice. Season fish with salt and pepper. Let marinate at room temperature for 10 minutes, turning fish to coat both sides.

Brush grill rack with oil. Grill fish until just opaque in center, about 5 minutes per side. Transfer to plates. Toss salsa gently and spoon strawberry-avocado salsa over fish. Squeeze a lime wedge over each fish and serve.

Tip: This dish works with other white fish like ono and mahi-mahi.

Salmon Fillets with Lemon and Garlic

SERVES: 4

16 ounces wild salmon fillet (four 4-ounce portions)

4 tablespoons extra-virgin olive oil

2 large lemons, sliced

Zest of 1 large lemon

3 cloves garlic, minced

1 teaspoon chopped thyme leaves

1 teaspoon dried oregano

1 teaspoon sea salt

Cracked black pepper, to taste

2 tablespoons finely chopped fresh parsley

Preheat oven to 400°F. Let salmon rest at room temperature. Line a large rimmed baking sheet with parchment paper and grease with olive oil. Place the lemon slices in an even layer. Season both sides of the salmon with salt and pepper and place on top of lemon slices.

In a small bowl, whisk together olive oil, lemon zest, garlic, thyme, and oregano. Rub mixture onto each piece of salmon by hand. Bake until the salmon is cooked through, about 25 minutes. Switch the oven to broil, and broil for 2 minutes, or until the olive oil/herb mixture has thickened slightly.

Garnish with parsley before serving.

Tip: Pair this dish with your favorite roasted vegetables, or my Sautéed Garlic Vegetables (recipe on page 340)

Healthy Italian Tuna Salad

MAKES 4 CUPS; SERVES: 4

Juice of 1 lemon

1 tablespoon capers, drained and chopped

¼ cup red onion, minced

1 teaspoon Dijon mustard

4 tablespoons fresh parsley, chopped finely

4 tablespoons extra-virgin olive oil

¼ teaspoon salt

⅛ teaspoon cracked black pepper

9 ounces cannellini beans, drained and rinsed

2 cans albacore tuna, in water, no salt added, drained

In a large glass bowl, mix together the lemon juice, capers, red onion, Dijon mustard, and fresh parsley. While continuing to mix, drizzle in the olive oil in a steady stream. Add in salt and pepper. Add the cannellini beans to the dressing and mash gently with a spoon. Add the tuna, breaking it up with a fork into bite-size pieces. Toss lightly to coat. Let sit for 30 minutes before serving. Serve on a bed of lettuce or arugula with sliced avocado.

Sautéed Shrimp with Lemon and Parsley

SERVES: 2

2 tablespoons extra-virgin olive oil, divided

4 cloves garlic, minced

10 ounces medium wild-caught shrimp, peeled and deveined (approximately 30 count)

Zest of one lemon

1 bunch fresh flat leaf parsley, chopped

Juice of 1 lemon

1–2 pinches sea salt and freshly cracked pepper

In a large sauté pan on medium-low heat, add enough olive oil to coat, about 1 1/2 tablespoons, and the cloves of minced garlic. Add the shrimp so they are all even on the bottom of the pan. Add lemon zest and season with sea salt and freshly ground pepper. Cook for 1 to 2 minutes and flip, until shrimp just begins to turn opaque. Add parsley, lemon juice, and 1/2 tablespoon of olive oil and mix together to coat the shrimp.

Serve hot on top of cooked spaghetti squash, or warm on a top of a fresh mix-and-match salad.

Turkey Meatballs with Spaghetti Squash and Cherry Tomato–Basil Sauce

SERVES: 4–6

FOR THE MEATBALLS

2 pounds lean ground turkey

3 garlic cloves, minced

¼ cup fresh parsley, chopped finely

⅛ teaspoon cumin

¼ teaspoon turmeric

½ teaspoon dried Italian herbs (premixed or use thyme, oregano, parsley, and basil)

⅛ teaspoon cracked black pepper

Small pinch sea salt

4 tablespoons extra-virgin olive oil

Preheat the oven to 350°F. Line a rimmed baking sheet with parchment paper.

In a large bowl, combine all of the ingredients. Mix well by hand until all ingredients are incorporated into the meat. Roll the meat mixture into golf-sized balls.

Place meatballs on the prepared baking sheet, leaving a little space between meatballs. Bake for 15–20 minutes, or until an internal thermometer reads 155°F for 15 seconds.

Italian Cherry Tomato–Basil Sauce

SERVES: 4–6

¼ cup olive oil

3 garlic cloves, minced

¼ cup onion, diced

4 cups cherry tomatoes, halved or quartered (2 pints)

1 teaspoon kosher salt

½ teaspoon fresh ground black pepper

¼ cup lightly packed fresh basil leaves, torn into small pieces

In a large skillet, heat the olive oil over medium heat. Add garlic and sauté 1 minute or until fragrant. Add the onion and sauté for 4–5 mins, or until starting to turn translucent, but not browned.

Add the cherry tomatoes, salt and pepper. As the tomatoes cook and soften, mash them lightly with a spatula or fork to create a chunky tomato sauce. Cook the tomatoes for approximately 6 minutes total.

Sprinkle with torn basil.

Transfer the tomato sauce to a bowl with cooked spaghetti squash, and toss to combine. To serve, add 3–4 turkey meatballs on top of spaghetti squash and serve warm.

Garnish with additional basil, if desired.

Tip: *Add cherry tomato sauce to roasted veggies for extra flavor.*
Note: *If you are not eating nightshades, substitute a pesto sauce for the cherry tomato sauce (recipe opposite).*

Creamy Zesty Pesto

MAKES ABOUT 2 CUPS; SERVES: 10–12
(1–2 TABLESPOONS PER SERVING)

¼ cup pine nuts or walnuts (if nut-free, try sunflower seeds!)

2 tablespoons nutritional yeast

2 garlic cloves, roughly chopped

2 cups packed fresh Italian basil, leaves torn from stem

1 teaspoon lemon zest

Juice of 1 lemon

½ cup extra-virgin olive oil

½ teaspoon sea salt

¼ teaspoon cracked black pepper

¼–½ cup filtered water (add more as needed)

In a small food processor, combine the pine nuts, nutritional yeast, garlic, basil, lemon zest, lemon juice, olive oil, salt, and pepper. Slowly drizzle in water while the processor is on until you get a slightly runny consistency to the pesto.

Chicken Fajitas with Cauliflower Rice

SERVING SIZE: $1/2$ CUP CAULIFLOWER RICE, $1/4$–$1/2$ CUP BLACK BEANS, 4–5 OUNCES CHICKEN PER PERSON, $1/2$ CUP VEGGIES, 2 TABLESPOONS DRESSING; SERVES: 4

1 ½ pounds boneless, skinless chicken thighs

1 teaspoon paprika

½ teaspoon ground cumin

1 teaspoon sea salt, divided

½ teaspoon cracked black pepper

2 tablespoons organic cold-pressed coconut oil, divided

2 bell peppers

1 yellow onion

2 medium zucchini

2 cups Cauliflower Rice (page 339)

| 1 15-ounce can black beans, rinsed and drained | Drizzle of Avocado Sauce or vinaigrette dressing of choice (pages 336–339) |
| 2 tablespoons cilantro, chopped | |

Preheat a large grill pan on medium to high heat. Meanwhile, season the chicken thighs in a large bowl with the paprika, cumin, $1/2$ teaspoon salt, and pepper. Spread 1 tablespoon coconut oil on a paper towel and wipe the grill pan to grease. Once hot, place the chicken thighs onto the pan. Cook 4–5 minutes on each side and remove, placing on a plate to rest.

Cut each bell pepper into $1/2$-inch-wide strips. Cut the onion in half, peel, and then cut one half into inch wide, reserving the other half. Cut the zucchini into $1/2$-inch-thick half moons. Toss the bell peppers, zucchini, and onion into the same grill pan, stirring every 2 to 3 minutes until softened through, a total of about 8 to 10 minutes. Turn heat off.

Meanwhile, preheat a medium saucepan on medium to high heat. Dice the remaining half of the onion. Add the remaining coconut oil and diced onion to the saucepan, stirring often. Once the onion has become translucent, about 3 to 4 minutes, add the cauliflower rice and black beans and sprinkle with remaining sea salt. Stir until heated through, about 4 to 5 minutes. Toss in the chopped cilantro and mix well. Turn heat off.

Slice the chicken thigh into long strips. Serve the cauliflower and black bean mixture onto plates, top with the grilled vegetables and chicken, then drizzle with your favorite vinaigrette dressing. I love the Avocado Sauce (page 316) or Creamy Green Goddess (page 338) for this recipe. Enjoy warm!

Tips: *Leftover cauliflower "rice" and beans can be enjoyed for breakfast. Make this dish vegetarian by substituting the chicken with a hearty vegetable or starch such as sweet potato.*

Add guacamole to this dish for a serving of healthy fats.

Easy Turkey Burger

SERVES: 4–5

I pound lean ground turkey

¼ cup red or white onion, minced

I teaspoon salt

¼ teaspoon black pepper

¼ teaspoon garlic powder

I teaspoon cumin

¼ cup packed fresh basil, chopped

¼ cup packed fresh parsley, chopped

I tablespoon extra-virgin olive oil

Lettuce wraps and your choice of toppings, including tomato, avocado, red onion, and pickles

In a large bowl, add the ground turkey meat, onion, salt, pepper, garlic powder, cumin, basil, and parsley. Mix and combine well with hands. Form into 4–5 turkey patties.

In a medium saucepan, heat the olive oil on medium-high and immediately add the patties. Cook for 5 minutes on each side. Serve on a lettuce wrap with toppings of your choice (tomato, avocado, red onion, and pickles).

Tips: *Consider adding Avocado Sauce or pesto to boost the flavor and add a fresh mix-and-match salad and sweet potato fries (page 341) for a complete meal.*

Consider using leftover patties for salads or on top of spaghetti squash for a quick and easy meal.

Hormone-Loving Bone Broth

MAKES 1½ GALLONS; SERVES: 12

I whole chicken carcass (a 3- to 7-pound whole chicken works well)

½ pound whole carrots (about 4 to 5 large carrots), rough chopped

½ head celery (about 4 to 5 stalks), rough chopped

I large yellow onion, peeled and quartered

3 bay leaves

½ bunch thyme

½ bunch parsley

4 garlic cloves, unpeeled

2-inch piece ginger, rough chopped

2 tablespoons apple cider vinegar

I tablespoon Himalayan pink salt or color rich salt (optional)

I gallon filtered water or enough to cover the carcass

2 teaspoons turmeric

Heat a large heavy-bottomed pot on high heat. Once the pot is hot, add the chicken carcass, backbone side down to brown the skin. Brown for about 2–3 minutes, then add the remaining ingredients except for the turmeric and pour in enough filtered water to cover the carcass. Bring to a rolling boil, cover, and lower heat to a simmer. Simmer on low for up to 24 hours, adding the turmeric in the last hour of cooking. Strain and discard all of the ingredients and separate into several glass jars for storage. Sip on its own in between meals or use in place of water for cooking quinoa.

Tip: *You can also make this bone broth in a slow cooker.*

Chard and White Bean Soup

SERVES: 6–8

2 tablespoons extra-virgin olive oil

3 medium carrots, sliced

3 celery stalks, sliced

1 large yellow onion, chopped

3 cloves garlic, minced

2 yellow zucchini, cubed

½ teaspoon dried oregano

⅛ teaspoon sea salt

1 quart low-sodium vegetable broth or Hormone-Loving Bone Broth (opposite)

3 sprigs fresh thyme, chopped

2 cups chard, rough chopped

1 can (9 ounces) cannellini beans, rinsed and drained

Heat the olive oil in a large pot over medium heat. Add the carrots, celery, onions, and garlic until they begin to soften, about 4–5 minutes. Add the zucchini, oregano, and sea salt; cook for 1 minute. Add the broth and thyme. Bring to a boil, then reduce heat, cover and simmer for an additional ten minutes. Then add the chard and beans and continue simmering until the chard is wilted and the carrots are soft, about 8–10 more minutes. Serve hot.

Creamy Chicken and Veggie Soup

This creamy, dairy-free chicken and veggie soup is one of my favorite comfort foods and it's easy to make. This soup is loaded up with lots of hearty veggies, chicken, fresh herbs, and a dash of creamy cashew cream, making it a creamy treat on cold nights.

SERVES: 6

FOR CASHEW CREAM

1 cup raw cashews

¾ cup just-boiled filtered water, plus more to soak cashews

Pinch of salt to taste

FOR CHICKEN AND VEGETABLE SOUP

¼ cup extra-virgin olive oil

1 medium-sized onion, diced

4–5 carrots, cut into rounds

4 stalks celery, thinly sliced

3 cloves garlic, chopped

1 teaspoon sea salt

1 tablespoon Italian seasoning

1 bay leaf

1.5 quarts bone, chicken, or vegetable broth

2 pounds boneless, skinless chicken breasts

3 cups packed baby spinach

¼ cup fresh Italian parsley, chopped

Salt and pepper, to taste

In a small heat-proof bowl, pour just-boiled water over the raw cashews and set aside to soak. Allow enough time for them to soak for at least 60 minutes. For preparation in advance, you can soak the cashews overnight, which is even better.

In a large soup pot, heat oil over medium heat with onions, carrots, celery, garlic, and sea salt.

Cook, stirring occasionally, for about 8–10 minutes, until soft and starting to caramelize.

Add Italian seasoning and bay leaf and continue to cook, stirring occasionally, for 1–2 minutes. Add broth and chicken breasts. Bring back up to a simmer.

Simmer for about 20–25 minutes, or until chicken is cooked through and veggies are tender.

Once the chicken is cooked, remove from the soup to a cutting board. Wait for it to cool slightly and then shred using two forks.

Prepare the cashew cream. Drain and rinse soaked cashews and add to a high-speed blender with about 1 cup of just-boiled water and pinch of salt.

Blend on high for a minute or two, until completely smooth and no pieces of cashew remain.

Add chicken back to the pot along with cashew cream and bring back to a simmer. Simmer for about 5–10 minutes to thicken the soup slightly.

Turn off the heat. Add baby spinach and stir until wilted.

Stir in fresh parsley, season to taste with salt and pepper, and serve warm!

Creamy Sweet Potato and Carrot Soup

SERVES: 6-8

2 tablespoons extra-virgin olive oil

1 large garlic clove, minced

¾ white onion, chopped

2 ½ liters low-sodium vegetable or bone broth

1 ½ pounds sweet potatoes (about 2 small), peeled and chopped into 1-inch pieces

4 large carrots, trimmed and cut into ¼-inch pieces

1 large Granny Smith apple, peeled, cored, and sliced

1-inch piece fresh ginger, peeled and sliced

½ tablespoon fresh thyme, chopped finely

1 tablespoon lemon juice

Freshly ground black pepper to taste

1 tablespoon fresh parsley, chopped

In a large pot, add the olive oil, garlic, and onion. Sauté a few minutes, until the onions have softened. Add the broth, sweet potatoes, carrots, apple, ginger, and thyme and bring to a boil over medium heat. Cook for 15–20 minutes or until the potatoes and carrots are very tender. Stir in lemon juice. Reduce heat and, in batches, transfer the entire soup contents to a blender. Blend soup on low to mix, then on high to smooth. Add black pepper, salt to taste. Sprinkle fresh parsley on top before serving.

Dressings

VINAIGRETTE DRESSINGS

Note: To create emulsions with these dressings, slowly add in olive oil while whisking vinegar. This is called emulsifying, which means that the oil and vinegar are becoming one because of the air bubbles created by the constant whisking, producing a thick mixture instead of separated oil and vinegar.

For oil-based vinaigrettes, follow this general rule of thumb:

1 part acid: 2 parts oil

1. Acid can be any of the vinegars from the Oils and Vinegars list (page 291) and lemon/lime juice.
2. Oil can be any of the oils from the Oils and Vinegars list (melt down coconut oil before using).
3. Always include mustard (mustard powder works, too!) as a thickener.

Example: 1 teaspoon Dijon mustard plus ½ cup vinegar plus 1 cup olive oil, slowly drizzled in while whisking. Finish with fresh chopped herbs, salt, and pepper to taste.

Simple Lemon Vinaigrette

MAKES ¾ CUP DRESSING; SERVES: 6

Juice of 3 lemons (about ¼ cup)

½ teaspoon lemon zest

⅛ teaspoon sea salt

⅛ teaspoon cracked black pepper

½ cup extra-virgin olive oil

Whisk together the lemon juice, lemon zest, salt, and pepper in a small bowl. Very slowly, drizzle in the olive oil and continue whisking the mixture together. Store in an airtight container or jar for future use.

Herbal Vinaigrette Dressing

MAKES 1 CUP DRESSING; SERVES: 6

½ cup loosely packed fresh parsley, roughly chopped

10 large fresh basil leaves

¼ teaspoon dried oregano

2 medium cloves garlic, roughly chopped

½ teaspoon Dijon mustard or brown mustard

¼ cup apple cider vinegar or red wine vinegar

¾ cup extra-virgin olive oil

⅛ teaspoon sea salt

Cracked black pepper, to taste

Combine the parsley, basil, oregano, garlic, mustard, and vinegar in the bowl of a food processor and process until a paste forms. With the machine running, drizzle in the olive oil to form an emulsion. Season to taste with salt and pepper. Vinaigrette is best used immediately, but can be stored in a sealed container in the refrigerator for up to 5 days.

Raspberry Lime Vinaigrette Dressing

MAKES 1 CUP DRESSING; SERVES: 6

1 cup raspberries, fresh or frozen

½ cup extra-virgin olive oil

¼ cup red wine vinegar

Juice of ¼ lime

½ teaspoon lime zest

⅛ teaspoon sea salt

Cracked black pepper, to taste

Place all of the ingredients in a blender and blend until smooth, adding water if too thick for your taste. Store in an airtight container or jar for up to a week in the fridge.

Creamy Green Goddess Dressing

MAKES 10-12 OUNCES

2 small to medium avocados

Juice of 1 large lime

¼ cup avocado or extra-virgin olive oil

⅓ cup filtered water

¾ cup packed basil leaves

¼ cup chopped parsley

¼ cup chopped scallions (approximately 2 scallions), white parts removed

2 tablespoons apple cider vinegar

Salt and white pepper, to taste

In a food processor or high-speed blender, blend all of the ingredients until smooth and creamy.

Store in an airtight mason jar (don't forget to label and date it!). Shake well before using. Keep in the refrigerator for three days max.

Tips: *This recipe is very flexible. Like more acid? Add more lime or lemon juice. Like the dressing runnier? Add more water.*

If you do not own a high-powered blender, a food processor will work, but the texture will not be as creamy.

Recipe twist: *For Latin-inspired dishes, substitute the majority of your herbs with cilantro, lemon for lime juice, and add half a seeded jalapeño and a pinch of ground cumin.*

Tahini Dressing

MAKES ABOUT 8 OUNCES; SERVES: 8-10

3 tablespoons tahini paste

½ cup filtered water

1 teaspoon olive oil

1 raw garlic clove

Juice of ½ medium lemon

Salt and pepper, to taste

In a food processor or high-speed blender, blend all the ingredients. If a runnier consistency is desired, simply add more water while blending.

Side Dishes

Cauliflower Rice

SERVES: 4

1 head cauliflower, washed

2 tablespoons extra-virgin olive oil

½ white onion, diced

Salt and pepper, to taste

Cut the cauliflower head in half and chop cauliflower into small florets so that the pieces will fit into a food processor. Insert the grater adapter into your food processor and start feeding the cauliflower florets through the top. Heat the olive oil in a large pan and sauté the diced onion until it's translucent. Add the cauliflower rice to the pan and sauté for another 5-7 minutes. Season with salt and pepper and serve immediately.

Dr. Mariza's Guacamole

SERVES: 4–6

6 avocados, pitted

½ cup cherry tomatoes, quartered

¼ cup white onion, chopped

¼ cup cilantro, chopped

Juice of 2 limes

¼ teaspoon garlic powder

½ teaspoon sea salt

½ teaspoon cracked black pepper

½ jalapeño or serrano chile, chopped finely (optional)

When pitting avocados, reserve two pits for later use. Scoop the flesh out of the avocados and put into a large bowl. Mash the avocados with a fork or potato masher to desired consistency. Add the remaining ingredients and mix well. Store guacamole with the two pits, to help slow the oxidation, or browning, process.

Sautéed Garlic Vegetables

SERVES: 4

2 tablespoons extra-virgin olive oil

¼ white onion, chopped

I large garlic clove, chopped

1 ½ cups cauliflower florets, thickly sliced

I green zucchini, sliced

I yellow bell pepper, sliced

I tablespoon fresh parsley, chopped

Juice of ½ lemon

Salt and pepper, to taste

Heat the olive oil in a large pan over medium heat. Add the onion and garlic and sauté for about a minute. Add the cauliflower florets and sauté for 2–3 minutes. Add the zucchini, bell pepper, fresh parsley, and lemon juice and cook for 4–5 more minutes. Remove from heat and season with salt and pepper to taste before serving.

Spaghetti Squash

SERVES: 2-4

1 spaghetti squash

1 teaspoon extra-virgin olive oil

Salt and pepper, to taste

Preheat the oven to 400°F. Cut the spaghetti squash in half lengthwise and scoop out the seeds. Drizzle both sides of the squash with olive oil and sprinkle with a pinch of salt and pepper. Place both sides of the spaghetti squash cut-side down on a baking sheet and use a fork to poke holes. Roast the spaghetti squash for 30 to 40 minutes or until the squash is lightly browned on the outside. The roasting time will depend on the size of the squash. Remove the squash from the oven and turn it over so that the cut side is up. Once it cools down, use a fork to scrape out the strands from the sides of the squash. Serve warm as a side.

Tip: *Top the squash with pesto or tomato sauce (recipes on page 328–329).*

Baked Sweet Potato Fries

SERVES: 3-4

2 large sweet potatoes (1 pound)

1 tablespoon extra-virgin olive oil

1 teaspoon dried oregano

1 teaspoon onion powder

1 teaspoon garlic powder

1 teaspoon ground cumin

1 teaspoon sweet paprika

¼ teaspoon cayenne pepper (optional)

½ teaspoon sea salt

⅛ teaspoon ground black pepper

Preheat the oven to 390°F.

Peel the sweet potato (optional) and cut it into sticks.

Place the sweet potato sticks and the rest of the ingredients in a large bowl and mix them until well combined. Spread the fries evenly on a parchment-lined baking sheet, making sure that they are not touching, which can result in soft fries. Bake fries for 15 minutes and then flip all the fries and bake for 10–15 more minutes, or until they are crispy and golden brown.

Salt and pepper them to taste and let them sit for 5 minutes. Enjoy warm!

Chapter 18

Day 22 and Beyond: Looking Back and to the Future

Congratulations! You did it. You've completed the 21-Day Hormone Makeover Program.

I know you are feeling more energized. Your skin is glowing, you've dropped a few pounds, you are hydrating daily and moving your body—and you are taking care of yourself. This is your new normal!

Day 22 Reflection Exercise

Now that your 21-Day Makeover is over, let's take a moment to evaluate what you've learned and how you want to go forward from here. What worked for you? Why? What do you want to continue doing in the days and months to come? Consider the following.

Go back to your Vision for Success exercise. Where did you see yourself ending up after our 21 days together? Did you achieve those goals? Where did you come up short? What exceeded your expectations? Evaluate your successes and stumbling blocks, and figure out where you want to dedicate more time to continue to see lasting change. You already know you can do it! Challenge yourself to continue your journey tomorrow. This is not the end; it's just the beginning.

Food Journal and Self-Care Journal. This is where you'll see tangible ways you have grown and changed over the last three weeks. In your food journal, look at what foods aided your body with energy, and acknowledge any that didn't serve your highest healing potential. In your Self-Care Journal, examine how your mood, stress, and relationships to self-care and food have changed. Look for patterns indicating the power of certain foods to empower your mood and vitality, as well as examples where it took away from your energy or focus. Reflecting on how far you have come can be your North Star in creating lasting success moving forward.

Check in with your body. Take a few minutes to just sit quietly. Close your eyes and listen to your body. Start with your head: Are you feeling like you can think more clearly? Are your brain fog or headaches gone? How about emotionally? Are you feeling more stable, optimistic, and empowered? Gradually move down your body and acknowledge the changes you've experienced over the last 21 days. Where have you seen the most change? What changes would you like to continue to foster in your life?

Identify three self-care rituals you want to continue. Whether it was the first time you spent dedicated time caring for yourself each day or if you've been in and out of a self-care routine, now is the time to identify the things that made your soul sing over the last three weeks and congratulate yourself for a job well done. Whether it's a new essential oil blend or nighttime wind-down ritual, allow yourself to prioritize these self-care rituals today and always.

What did you love about the program? What would you change? Taking time to evaluate the experience you just committed the last three weeks of your life to will ensure you can look back with appreciation and optimism regarding how far you have come. Be honest with yourself. If it didn't work for you, that's okay. I invite you to try the Hormone Makeover again, knowing what you know now to make it work better for you this time.

What's Next?

After you complete this exercise, it's time to create a plan for your future. This is what we call reentry. Now that you know you can have an established routine of amazing healing habits, maintaining them and continuing to move forward with your success is your goal. But it's also important to create a plan so you don't fall back into old habits that sabotage all the gains you've made.

Can you continue the 21-Day Program for another 7, 14, or even 21 days? Absolutely you can! I have personally stayed on this program for 90 days at a time. It will continue to provide you with amazing results, even more than the first 21 days. These recipes, supplement protocols, and self-care guides have been created to integrate easily into your everyday life so much so that you can continue this plan indefinitely if you choose to do so. Even more amazing is the power you have found in implementing the program in your life, knowing that the longer you continue, the more habitual it will become. Soon you will find that you don't even have to think about the particulars, but that you have effectively transformed your life. But even better yet, now that you have the basics of this healing program under your belt, you can customize it even more to continue your individual long-term success.

How to Measure Your Continued Progress

Take your numbers and measurements again to assess any changes. More important, take a good look at yourself in the mirror. Note any changes to your skin tone, hair texture, the way you look and feel in your clothes, the smile you give yourself when you see your success in such a physical way, or just your overall sense of self. Appreciating and loving what you see in the mirror matters. *This* is more important than a number any day of the week.

Reentry Planning

Each of the tenets we've covered in the 21-Day Makeover has the potential to easily integrate into your "normal life" routines. Before we get into some specifics, answer this question: What do you want your new normal to be? Now is the perfect time to set your ambitions higher than you ever believed possible. You don't have to go back to the hot flashes, fatigue, poor digestion, lagging libido, or extra weight. *This* can be your normal!

Here are some simple tips in each of the categories we've focused on to help you get back to your normal life while still sustaining the progress you've made.

Leverage Your Food Journal

Analyze your Food Journal to determine what foods you loved to eat and what you could do without. More important, figure out what foods affect your body and your mood after each meal. In the future, use it to track your whole foods and individualized meal plan. Your shopping lists should still be whole foods that you can cook and prepare on your own as much as possible. Stick to the Yes/No foods list in the future, which are essential to create and maintain success. You can begin to reintroduce foods (see below), but be mindful and proceed with caution. There is nothing wrong with sticking to the meal plan and adding your own recipes with the knowledge you've gained. If you move away from the meal plan, be mindful of portion control and continue to support your body with foods that heal your body, especially green smoothies with quality protein powder, fiber, and superfoods!

Use the 1-2-3 Rule to Reintroduce Foods

If you decide you do want to reintroduce some foods you had removed, you need to be patient and start slowly. Don't add them all back at the same time, even if it is just a little bit. Choose one food and then eat it once, waiting one day afterward while recording how your body responds. Then eat it twice in one day, waiting another two days and recording the results. Then eat it three times in one day and wait three days. Jot down in your Food Journal what you notice, from mood, to digestion, to bowel movements. Continue to pay attention for the first couple of weeks, as you may not have a symptom until the food builds back up in your system. After those three days are over and you decide whether or not your body is accepting this food back into your daily routines, you can repeat the process with the next food. Reintroduce the foods in the following order: red meat, dairy, grains, gluten, sugar, caffeine, and nightshades (if you remove them).

If you know you have an autoimmune condition or a chronic condition that is impacted by highly inflammatory foods, consider removing gluten, dairy, and excess sugar entirely. I can speak from experience that these three food groups increase inflammation and can deregulate hormone pathways.

Keep Hydrating Daily

Even if water infusions weren't for you, your body needs to stay hydrated. Keep playing around with fruit or vegetable infusions to find the ones you love. Do whatever you need to do to keep up your water intake! Tracking your water intake with an app also helps you be really aware of your hydration levels. I recommend trying this for a while until it becomes routine for you.

Continue with Green Smoothies

I have had a green smoothie for breakfast every day for years, and my body has never felt better. This is the best way to set yourself up for all-day success! Now that you have the basics down, have fun with it! Just remember to always include plenty of leafy greens and healthy fruits or vegetables, healthy fat, protein powder, and fiber to make it a complete meal.

Stick with Supplements

Continue with the Foundational Daily Hormone Support Protocol to maintain your results. If you added a specific protocol (such as for thyroid, gut, liver, stress, mood, or insulin balance) and you feel like you still want to continue making gains in that area, keep going with that protocol for another few weeks, then reevaluate again. Or, if you feel the supplements aren't working for you and you want to press pause to see how your body responds, go ahead. Use your daily journaling to track your body's response. (And I don't recommend changing supplementation while reintroducing foods!)

Practice Self-Care Routines and Rituals with Essential Oils

I urge you to continue your self-care routines and rituals. Be mindful about living with intent and purpose. Practice gratitude journaling. Spread love. Take time when you eat. Appreciate the beauty around you. Continue to use your essential oils, especially the blends that you love.

Continue Your Daily Movement

Exercise is *so* important for women in our stage of life. As you enter your thirties, forties, fifties, and beyond, it's okay if your movement practices evolve and change to suit your needs. Be in tune with what feels good and what is causing unnecessary stress. But no matter what, keep moving your body!

Reduce Your Toxic Load

Continue to make hormone-loving choices with your personal and beauty care products, cleaning products, and anything that you put on or in your body. Control what you can in your environment by cleaning regularly and airing out your home. Use the Environmental

Working Group's website to check any new products you are considering, and check out my bestselling book *Smart Mom's Guide to Essential Oils* for amazing DIY products and guides.

Set Boundaries

Be smart about life events like birthday parties and holidays. Know your trigger foods and plan accordingly. Eat before events, pack your own snacks, carry your water, and bring along an accountability partner. And consider the effect of toxic people on your energy. If they aren't building you up, they are absolutely tearing you down. Create some distance, and see how you feel. It's all about what is best for you and your health, and anything that creates stress impedes your progress.

Most Important, Give Yourself the Credit That You Deserve

You did a fantastic job over the last three weeks! Take a moment to acknowledge that and keep coming back to that feeling each and every day moving forward. Know that *self-care is healthcare* and you are the CEO of your own healthcare. Self-care is not selfish, and you do *not* need to feel any guilt about it. It helps you nourish your own body, mind, and soul so that you can be your best self possible and give the world the best of you.

Now that you are entering the next phase, I am thrilled to continue this journey with you and to provide you with more support and resources. Please continue to count on me as your guide as you navigate midlife with confidence and grace. I have curated an amazing midlife toolkit for you that includes delicious recipes, quick how-to videos, cheat sheets, and expert interviews. You can find your toolkit at www.drmariza.com/toolkit.

No matter where you are in your journey, imagine me and a community of women cheering you on each day. I am so proud of you for making a commitment to yourself and your health. And I am confident that, with the tools and resources in this book, you will continue to make choices that serve your highest good. You have so much to give this world and when you feel energized and empowered, you are unstoppable.

Lastly, I want to invite you to explore passions and activities that bring you joy! Consider creating a joy list and integrate things you love into your every day. Ask yourself each morning, "What would I love?" and see what inspires you.

This new phase in your life is going to open new doors and provide new perspectives. I know for a fact that you are a positive influence in this world. By choosing to show up with joy and positive energy, you will be more receptive to endless creative possibilities. It's time to embrace those creative possibilities and shine your bright light everywhere you go.

Selected Bibliography

The following citations represent the main sources of my research. For a complete listing of all sources, please visit www.drmariza .com/bibliography.

Agnoli, A., V. Andreoli, M. Casacchia, and R. Cerbo. 1976. "Effect of S-adenosyl-{l}-methionine (SAMe) upon Depressive Symptoms." *Journal of Psychiatric Research* 13, no. 1: 43–54. https://doi.org/10.1016/0022-3956(76)90008-X.

Aguilar, M., T. Bhuket, S. Torres, B. Liu, and R. J. Wong. 2015. "Prevalence of the Metabolic Syndrome in the United States, 2003–2012." *Journal of the American Medical Association* 313, no. 19: 1973. https://doi.org/10.1001/jama .2015.4260.

Andersen, M. L., R. A. Bittencourt, I. B. Antunes, and S. Tufik. 2006. "Effects of Progesterone on Sleep: A Possible Pharmacological Treatment for Sleep-Breathing Disorders?" *Current Medicinal Chemistry* 13, no. 29: 3575–82. https://doi.org/10.2174/092986706779026200.

Ayers, B., M. Forshaw, and M. S. Hunter. 2010. "The Impact of Attitudes Towards the Menopause on Women's Symptom Experience: A Systematic Review." *Maturitas* 65, no. 1: 28–36. https://doi.org/10.1016/j.maturitas.2009.10.016.

Boneva, R. S., J. M. Lin, and E. R. Unger. 2015. "Early Menopause and Other Gynecologic Risk Indicators for Chronic Fatigue Syndrome in Women." *Menopause* 22, no. 8: 826–34. https://doi.org/10.1097/GME.0000000000000411.

Born, L., G. Koren, E. Lin, and M. Steiner. 2008. "A New, Female-Specific Irritability Rating Scale." *Journal of Psychiatry and Neuroscience: JPN* 33, no. 4: 344–54. PMID: 18592028.

Breus, Michael J. 2019. "3 Amazing Benefits of GABA." *Psychology Today.* https://www.psychologytoday.com/us/blog/sleep-newzzz/201901/3 -amazing-benefits-gaba.

Brown, R., P. L. Gerbarg, and Z. Ramazanov. "Rhodiola rosea: A Phytomedicinal Overview." http://www.medref.se/rosenrot/Brown_Rhodiola_rosea.pdf.

Caliceti, C., P. Rizzo, and A. Cicero. 2015. "Potential Benefits of Berberine in the Management of Perimenopausal Syndrome." *Oxidative Medicine and Cellular Longevity* no. 1: 1–9. https://doi.org/10.1155/2015/723093.

Calsolaro, V., G. Pasqualetti, F. Niccolai, et al. 2017. "Thyroid Disrupting Chemicals." *International Journal of Molecular Sciences* 18, no. 12: 2583. https://doi.org/10.3390/ijms18122583.

Castaneda, Ruben. 2018. "Why Many Women Unnecessarily Get a Hysterectomy." *U.S. News & World Report.* https://health.usnews.com/health-care/patient-advice/articles/2018-01-18/why-many-women-unnecessarily-get-a-hysterectomy.

Christie, A. D., E. Seery, and J. A. Kent. 2016. "Physical Activity, Sleep Quality, and Self-Reported Fatigue Across the Adult Lifespan." *Experimental Gerontology* 77: 7–11. https://doi.org/10.1016/j.exger.2016.02.001.

Clarke, G., R. M. Stilling, P. J. Kennedy, et al. 2014. "Gut Microbiota: The Neglected Endocrine Organ." *Molecular Endocrinology* 28, no. 8: 1221–38. https://doi.org/10.1210/me.2014-1108.

Daher, R., T. Yazbeck, J. B. Jaoude, and B. Abboud. 2009. "Consequences of Dysthyroidism on the Digestive Tract and Viscera." *World Journal of Gastroenterology* 15, no. 23: 2834–38. https://doi.org/10.3748/wjg.15.2834.

Dalal, P. K., and M. Agarwal. 2015. "Postmenopausal Syndrome." *Indian Journal of Psychiatry* 57, suppl. 2: S222–S232. https://doi.org/10.4103/0019-5545.161483.

Dienes K. A., N. A. Hazel, and C. L. Hammen. 2013. "Cortisol Secretion in Depressed and At-Risk Adults." *Psychoneuroendocrinology* 38, no. 6: 927–40. doi:10.1016/j.psyneuen.2012.09.019.

Domingo, S., and A. Pellicer. 2009. "Overview of Current Trends in Hysterectomy." *Expert Review of Obstetrics and Gynecology* 4, no. 6: 673–85. doi: 10.1586/eog.09.51.

Epperson, C. N., M. D. Sammel, T. L. Bale, et al. 2017. "Adverse Childhood Experiences and Risk for First-Episode Major Depression During the Menopause Transition." *Journal of Clinical Psychiatry* 78, no. 3: e298–e307. https://doi.org/10.4088/JCP.16m10662.

Fallahi, P., S. M. Ferrari, G. Elia, et al. 2018. "Myo-inositol in Autoimmune Thyroiditis, and Hypothyroidism." *Reviews in Endocrine and Metabolic Disorders* 19, no. 4: 349–54. https://doi.org/10.1007/s11154-018-9477-9.

Filler, K., D. Lyon, J. Bennett, N. McCain, et al. 2014. "Association of Mitochondrial Dysfunction and Fatigue: A Review of the Literature." *BBA Clinical* 1: 12–23. https://doi.org/10.1016/j.bbacli.2014.04.001.

Freedman, R., and T. Roehrs. 2007. "Sleep Disturbance in Menopause." *Menopause* 14, no. 5: 826–29. https://doi.org/10.1097/gme.0b013e3180321a22.

Gartoulla, P., R. Worsley, R. J. Bell, and S. R. Davis. 2015. "Moderate to Severe Vasomotor and Sexual Symptoms Remain Problematic for Women Aged

60 to 65 Years." *Menopause* 22, no. 7: 694–701. https://doi.org/10.1097/GME.0000000000000383.

Glade, M. J., and K. Smith. 2015. "Phosphatidylserine and the Human Brain." *Nutrition* 31, no. 6: 781–86. https://doi.org/10.1016/j.nut.2014.10.014.

Golbidi, S., M. Badran, and I. Laher. 2011. "Diabetes and Alpha Lipoic Acid." *Frontiers in Pharmacology* 2: 69. https://doi.org/10.3389/fphar.2011.00069.

Grady, D., and G. F. Sawaya. 2005. "Discontinuation of Postmenopausal Hormone Therapy." *American Journal of Medicine* 118, no. 12, supp. 2: 163–65. https://doi.org/10.1016/j.amjmed.2005.09.051.

Harvard Health Publishing, Harvard Medical School. 2019. "The Lowdown on Thyroid Slowdown." https://www.health.harvard.edu/diseases-and-conditions/the-lowdown-on-thyroid-slowdown.

Howell, A. B., and B. Foxman. 2002. "Cranberry Juice and Adhesion of Antibiotic-Resistant Uropathogens." *JAMA* 287, no. 23: 3082–83. https://doi.org/10.1001/jama.287.23.3082.

Hu, M. L., C. K. Rayner, K. L. Wu, et al. 2011. "Effect of Ginger on Gastric Motility and Symptoms of Functional Dyspepsia." *World Journal of Gastroenterology* 17, no. 1: 105–10. https://doi.org/10.3748/wjg.v17.i1.105.

Hunter, M., and M. Rendall. 2007. "Bio-psycho-socio-cultural Perspectives on Menopause." *Best Practice & Research Clinical Obstetrics and Gynaecology* 21, no. 2: 261–74. https://doi.org/10.1016/j.bpobgyn.2006.11.001.

Jokar, T. O, L. T. Fourman, H. Lee, et al. 2018. "Higher TSH Levels Within the Normal Range Are Associated with Unexplained Infertility." *Journal of Clinical Endocrinology & Metabolism* 103, no. 2: 632–39. https://doi.org/10.1210/jc.2017-02120.

Jones, R. K. 2011. "Beyond Birth Control: The Overlooked Benefits of Oral Contraceptive Pills." New York: Guttmacher Institute. https://www.guttmacher.org/sites/default/files/report_pdf/beyond-birth-control.pdf.

Kashefi, F., M. Khajehei, M. Alavinia, et al. 2015. "Effect of Ginger (*Zingiber officinale*) on Heavy Menstrual Bleeding: A Placebo-Controlled, Randomized Clinical Trial." *Phytotherapy Research: PTR* 29, no. 1: 114–19. https://doi.org/10.1002/ptr.5235.

Katz, T. A., Y. Qiwei, S. Treviño, et al. 2016. "Endocrine-Disrupting Chemicals and Uterine Fibroids." *Fertility and Sterility* 106, no. 4: 967–77. https://doi.org/10.1016/j.fertnstert.2016.08.023.

Kumar, V., R. Chodankar, and J. K. Gupta. 2016. "Endometrial Ablation for Heavy Menstrual Bleeding." *Women's Health (London)* 12, no. 1 (Jan.): 45–52. https://doi.org/10.2217/whe.15.86.

Lauritano, E. C., A. L. Bilotta, M. Gabrielli, et al. 2007. "Association Between Hypothyroidism and Small Intestinal Bacterial Overgrowth." *Journal of Clinical Endocrinology & Metabolism* 92, no. 11: 4180–84. https://doi.org/10.1210/jc.2007-0606.

Licznerska, B. E., H. Szaefer, M. Murias, et al. 2013. "Modulation of *CYP19* Expression by Cabbage Juices and Their Active Components: Indole-

3-carbinol and 3,3′-diindolylmethene in Human Breast Epithelial Cell Lines." *European Journal of Nutrition* 52: 1483–92. https://doi.org/10.1007/s00394-012-0455-9.

Manson, J. E., and A. M. Kaunitz. 2016. "Menopause Management—Getting Clinical Care Back on Track." *New England Journal of Medicine* 374: 803–6. https://doi.org/10.1056/NEJMp1514242.

Mao, J. J., S. X. Xie, J. Zee, et al. 2015. "Rhodiola rosea Versus Sertraline for Major Depressive Disorder: A Randomized Placebo-Controlled Trial." *Phytomedicine* 22, no. 3: 394–99. https://doi.org/10.1016/j.phymed.2015.01.010.

Mackawy, A. M. H., B. M. Al-Ayed, and B. M. Al-Rashidi. 2013. "Vitamin D Deficiency and Its Association with Thyroid Disease." *International Journal of Health Sciences* 7, no. 3: 267–75. https://doi.org/10.12816/0006054.

Mishra, S., and K. Palanivelu. 2008. "The Effect of Curcumin (Turmeric) on Alzheimer's Disease: An Overview." *Annals of Indian Academy of Neurology* 11, no. 1: 13–19. https://doi.org/10.4103/0972-2327.40220.

Mullaicharam, A. R. 2014. "A Review on Evidence Based Practice of *Ginkgo biloba* in Brain Health." *International Journal of Chemical and Pharmaceutical Analysis* 1, no. 1: 24–30.

National Center for Complementary and Integrative Health. 2017. "St. John's Wort and Depression: In Depth.". https://www.nccih.nih.gov/health/st-johns-wort-and-depression-in-depth.

Nouveau, S., P. Bastien, F. Baldo, and O. de Lacharriere. 2008. "Effects of Topical DHEA on Aging Skin: A Pilot Study." *Maturitas* 59, no. 2: 174–81. https://doi.org/10.1016/j.maturitas.2007.12.004.

Nygaard, I., M. D. Barber, K. L. Burgio, et al. 2008. "Prevalence of Symptomatic Pelvic Floor Disorders in U.S. Women." *JAMA* 300, no. 11: 1311–16. https://doi.org/10.1001/jama.300.11.1311.

Oyelowo, Tolu. 2007. "Menorrhagia." In *Mosby's Guide to Women's Health.* St. Louis, Missouri: Mosby Elsevier. https://doi.org/10.1016/B978-0-323-04601-5.X5001-1.

Palacios S., V. W. Henderson, N. Siseles, et al. 2010. "Age of Menopause and Impact of Climacteric Symptoms by Geographical Region." *Climacteric* 13, no. 5: 419–28. https://doi.org/10.3109/13697137.2010.507886.

Pulipati, S., P. S. Babu, M. L. Narasu, and N. Anusha. 2017. "An Overview on Urinary Tract Infections and Effective Natural Remedies." *Journal of Medicinal Plants Studies* 5, no. 6: 50–56. http://www.plantsjournal.com/archives/2017/vol5issue6/PartA/5-6-7-566.pdf.

Pyykkönen, A. J., B. Isomaa, A. K. Pesonen, J. G. Eriksson, et al. 2012. "Subjective Sleep Complaints Are Associated with Insulin Resistance in Individuals Without Diabetes: The PPP-Botnia Study." *Diabetes Care* 35, no. 11: 2271–78. https://doi.org/10.2337/dc12-0348.

Saaresranta, T., U. Anttalainen, and O. Polo. 2015. "Sleep Disordered Breathing: Is It Different for Females?" *ERJ Open Research* 1, no. 2: 00063-2015. https://doi.org/10.1183/23120541.00063-2015.

Saccomani, S., J. F. Lui-Filho, C. R. Juliato, et al. 2017. "Does Obesity Increase the Risk of Hot Flashes Among Midlife Women?: A Population-Based Study." *Menopause* 24, no. 9: 1065–70. https://doi.org/10.1097/GME.0000000000000884.

Secades, J. J., and J. L. Lorenzo. 2006. "Citicoline: Pharmacological and Clinical Review, 2006 Update." *Methods and Findings in Experimental and Clinical Pharmacology* 28, Suppl. B:1–56. PMID: 17171187.

Severo, J. S., J. Morais, T. de Freitas, et al. 2019. "The Role of Zinc in Thyroid Hormones Metabolism." *International Journal for Vitamin and Nutrition Research* 89, no. 1–2: 80–88. https://doi.org/10.1024/0300-9831/a000262.

Sharma, S., and N. Aggarwal. 2017. "Vitamin D and Pelvic Floor Disorders." *Journal of Mid-Life Health* 8, no. 3: 101–2. https://doi.org/10.4103/jmh.JMH_88_17.

Shoskes, D. A., and J. C. Nickel. 2011. "Quercetin for Chronic Prostatitis/Chronic Pelvic Pain Syndrome." *Urologic Clinics of North America* 38, no. 3: 279–84. https://doi.org/10.1016/j.ucl.2011.05.003.

Siegel, A. M., and S. B. Mathews. 2015. "Diagnosis and Treatment of Anxiety in the Aging Woman." *Current Psychiatry Reports* 17, no. 12: 93. https://doi.org/10.1007/s11920-015-0636-3.

Stewart, E. A., L. T. Shuster, and W. A Rocca. 2012. "Reassessing Hysterectomy." *Minnesota Medicine* 95, no. 3: 36–39. PMID: 22611818.

Thurston, R. C. 2013. "Cognition and the Menopausal Transition: Is Perception Reality?" *Menopause* 20, no. 12: 1231–32. https://doi.org/10.1097/GME.0000000000000137.

Tuomikoski, P., O. Ylikorkala, and T. S. Mikkola. 2012. "Menopausal Hot Flashes and Insulin Resistance." *Menopause* 19, no. 10: 1116–20. https://doi.org/10.1097/gme.0b013e3182503d5d.

Vahratian, A. 2017. "Sleep Duration and Quality Among Women Aged 40–59, by Menopausal Status." NCHS data brief no. 286. Hyattsville, MD: National Center for Health Statistics. https://www.cdc.gov/nchs/products/databriefs/db286.htm.

Ventura, M., M. Melo, and F. Carrilho. 2017. "Selenium and Thyroid Disease: From Pathophysiology to Treatment." *International Journal of Endocrinology* 2017: 1297658. https://doi.org/10.1155/2017/1297658.

Vollmer, G., A. Papke, and O. Zierau. 2010. "Treatment of Menopausal Symptoms by an Extract from the Roots of Rhapontic Rhubarb: The Role of Estrogen Receptors." *Chinese Medicine* 5: 7. https://doi.org/10.1186/1749-8546-5-7.

Wolburg, H., and A. Lippoldt. 2002. "Tight Junctions of the Blood-Brain Barrier: Development, Composition and Regulation." *Vascular Pharmacology* 38, no. 6: 323–37. https://doi.org/10.1016/S1537-1891(02)00200-8.

Wurtman, R. J., M. Regan, I. Ulus, and L. Yu. 2000. "Effect of Oral CDP-choline on Plasma Choline and Uridine Levels in Humans." *Biochemical Pharmacology* 60, no. 7: 989–92. https://doi.org/10.1016/s0006-2952(00)00436-6.

Wang, S., C. Zhang, G. Yang, and Y. Yang. 2014. "Biological Properties of 6-gingerol: A Brief Review." *Natural Product Communications* 9, no. 7: 1027–30. PMID: 25230520.

Wu, Y., Y. Zhang, G. Xie, et al. 2012. "The Metabolic Responses to Aerial Diffusion of Essential Oils." *PLoS One* 7, no. 9: e44830. https://doi.org/10.1371/journal.pone.0044830.

Xie, L., H. Kang, Q. Xu, et al. 2013. "Sleep Drives Metabolite Clearance from the Adult Brain." *Science* 342, no. 6156: 373–77. https://doi.org/10.1126/science.1241224.

Zhou, J., J. Y. Ko, S. C. Haight, and V. T. Tong. 2019. "Treatment of Substance Use Disorders Among Women of Reproductive Age by Depression and Anxiety Disorder Status, 2008–2014." *Journal of Women's Health (2002)* 28, no. 8: 1068–76. https://doi.org/10.1089/jwh.2018.7597.

Ziaei, S., A. Kazemnejad, and M. Zareai. 2007. "The Effect of Vitamin E on Hot Flashes in Menopausal Women." *Gynecologic and Obstetric Investigation* 64, no. 4: 204–7. https://doi.org/10.1159/000106491.

Zou, J., B. Chassaing, V. Singh, et al. 2017. "Fiber-Mediated Nourishment of Gut Microbiota Protects Against Diet-Induced Obesity by Restoring IL-22-Mediated Colonic Health." *Cell and Host Microbe* 23, no. 1: 41–53. https://doi.org/10.1016/j.chom.2017.11.003.

Resources

The following is a list of key resources to support your journey toward hormone balance and becoming the CEO of your health with self-care rituals, supplementation, and essential oils. For more inspiration, I have created an amazing midlife toolkit for you that includes delicious recipes, quick how-to videos, cheat sheets, and expert interviews. You can find your toolkit at www.drmariza.com/toolkit.

Quiz: What Is Causing Perimenopause and Menopause Hormonal Imbalances?
www.drmariza.com/quiz

Essentially Whole® Supplements for Perimenopause and Menopause
www.drmariza.com/store

Dr. Mariza's Daily Self-Care Journal
www.drmariza.com/journal

Hormone Testing and Trusted Laboratories
www.drmariza.com/labtests
https://dutchtest.com

Recommended High-Quality Essential Oils
www.drmariza.com/essentialoils

Getting Started with Essential Oils Checklist
www.drmariza.com/checklist

Essential Oil Accessories (Diffusers, Cases, Containers, Carrier Oils)
www.oillife.com
www.aromatools.com

Integrative and Functional Practitioners
https://www.ifm.org/find-a-practitioner/

Dr. Mariza's Go-To Experts
You can find many of these experts on the *Essentially You* podcast on
    iTunes.

Menopause and Hormone Support
Christiane Northrup, MD (https://www.drnorthrup.com)
Anna Cabeca, DO OBGYN (https://drannacabeca.com)
Dr. Taz, MD (https://doctortaz.com)
Bridgit Danner, LAC (http://www.bridgitdanner.com)
Sara Gottfried, MD (http://www.saragottfriedmd.com)
Alan Christianson, NMD (https://drchristianson.com)
Lara Briden, ND (https://www.larabriden.com)

Thyroid Support
Izabella Wentz, PharmaD, FASCP (www.thyroidpharmacist.com)
Magdalena Wszelaki (www.hormonesbalance.com)

Autoimmune Support
Amy Myers, MD (https://www.amymyersmd.com)
Tom O'Bryan, DC, CCN, DACBN (http://thedr.com)
Terry Wahls, MD (https://terrywahls.com)

Gut Support
Vincent Pedre, MD (http://pedremd.com)
Summer Bock, CNS (https://summerbock.com)

Nutrition Support
JJ Virgin, CNS, CHFS (https://jjvirgin.com)
Kellyann Petrucci, MS, ND (https://www.drkellyann.com)
Dave Asprey (https://www.bulletproof.com)
Stephanie Estima, DC (https://www.drstephanieestima.com)

Mindset and Emotional Support
Jennifer Hudye (https://www.visionvortex.com)
Trudy Scott, CN (http://www.antianxietyfoodsolution.com)
Kelly Brogan, MD (http://kellybroganmd.com)
Emily Fletcher (https://zivameditation.com)

Thank You!

I want to thank the following people for supporting me in writing this book and getting it out into the world to serve beautiful, amazing women.

Alex Dunks, my incredible husband, for going above and beyond during the countless months of writing this book. You are my favorite person in the world!

My beautiful mom, Jody DeLeone, for allowing me to share your story and for inspiring me to always reach for my dreams.

My grandmothers, Rachel Anguiano and Sharon Snyder, for your unwavering support.

To my readers: I am so grateful to you for allowing me to be a part of your healing journey. You are the reason I wrote this book.

Tami, Erin, Rebecca, Kristen, Jan, Caurel, Anne, Isabela, and the rest of my rock star team behind the scenes. I am so grateful for your passion and commitment to our mission.

To my incredible wolfpack: Jennifer Hudye, Amber Spears, Alona Rudnitsky, and Alex Moscow for being by my side through thick and thin and for always being down to celebrate all the wins.

JJ Virgin, for being a powerful inspiration, mentor, and friend. Bridgit Danner, for our weekly phone calls. Gabrielle Lyon, for taking care of me with love. Candace Romero, for having my back since I was twenty-two years old and always keeping it real.

To all of my fellow wellness rock stars: Stephanie Estima, Anna Cabeca, Elisa Song, Bree Argetsinger, Elena Brower, Vivian Glyck, Lisa Sasevich, Cleopatra Kamperveen, Joan Rosenberg, Amy Medling, Debra Atkinson, Izabella and Michael Wentz, Isa Herrera, Ari Whitten, Samantha Gladish, Melissa Esguerra, Nicole Jardim, McCall McPherson, Lauren Noel, Alan Christianson, Melissa Kathryn, Vincent Pedre, Dave Asprey, Teri Cochrane, Emily Fletcher, Alexandra Jamieson, Ann Shippy, Kevin and Annmarie Gianni, Zia Nicks, Brianne Hovey, Christiana Maia, Cynthia Pasquela, Summer Bock, Kellyann Petrucci, Jessica Drummond, Lisa Hendrickson-Jack, Amy Myers, Maru Davila, Nat Kringoudis, Shawn Tassone, Robyn Benson, Will Cole, Lara Adler, and Tricia Nelson—together we are changing the world!

My incredible publishing team—Wendy Sherman, thank you for being the best literary agent and believing in me every step of the way.

Julia Pastore, Erin Hubbard, and Rebecca Grow for helping me create this book and making it approachable for my readers.

Anna Z. Bohbot for being my fellow collaborator in all of my books and for creating incredible, healthy recipes.

The wonderful team at Rodale for partnering with me to create this book—Marnie Cochran, Christina Foxley, Odette Fleming, and all of the rock stars in the copyediting department.

Index

Note: Page numbers in parentheses indicate intermittent references. Page numbers in *italics* indicate essential oil blends.

pelvic floor dysfunction, urinary incontinence/UTIs (*cont.*)
supplements/herbal remedies for, 224–25, 228–29
support for, 222–29
urinary tract incontinence and UTIs, 217, 219–20, 226–29
what's going on, 217–20
why it's happening, 220–21
Pelvic Pain Massage Blend, *223*
Pelvic Soothe Relaxation Rollerball Blend, *223*
Pelvic Soothe Rollerball Blend, *242–43*
Pelvic Support Bath Soak, *224*
Peppermint essential oil, 50, 58, **68**, *70, 84, 85, 87, 102*, 109, 116, *117, 124*, (*131–33*), *164, 165, 178, 179*, 182, (*193–95*), *209*, 224, 231, *242*, 266
perimenopause. *See also specific topics*
defined, 16, 23
essential oils for, 69
hormone fluctuations, 16–17
hormones during, 29
mom's story, 4–6, 9
options for easing through, 17–19
symptoms and reality of, 16–17
Personal Inhaler Blends, *101*
personal inhalers and blends
about: inhaling essential oils, 55; personal inhalers, 64
for brain fog/cognitive function, *194*
for low energy/fatigue, *132*
for mood support, *149*
for sleep, *101–2*
for stress, *83*
Personal Sensuality Bath Soak, *210–11*
phytoestrogen boost routine, 120–21
phytoestrogens, 25, 32. *See also* dong quai
Pickled Red Onion, 321–22
planning meals, 281–82, 293–302. *See also* recipes *references*
plant-focused nutrition, benefits overview, 6
postmenopause, 22–23, 202, 236. *See also* menopause
progesterone. *See also* heavy bleeding and fibroids
bioidentical, 122, 247
brain fog/function and, 186, 189
digestive issues and, 170, 173

estrogen dominance and, 30–31, 125, 237
fertility phases and, (27–29)
hot flashes, night sweats and, 114–15
HRT and, 31–33
menopause and, 30
mood swings and, 143, 144
production and functions, 26
sleep and, 95–96, 97
stress and, 144, 238
synthetic, 18–19, 122, 250
thyroid issues and, 97, 240–41
protocols. *See also* Dr. Mariza's Hormone-Loving Rituals and Protocols

quiz, hormone, 47

Raspberry Lime Vinaigrette Dressing, 337
reactions vs. allergies/sensitivities, 66
recipes, about, 303
recipes, beverages/teas, 303–7. *See also* recipes, breakfast smoothies/shakes
about: digestive teas, 183; ginseng tea for hot flashes, 121; overview of, 303; uva-ursi tea, 229
Adrenal Love Tulsi Tea, 305–6
Chamomile/Passionflower/Lavender Tea, 105
Detox and Recharge Water Infusion, *89–90*
Iced Matcha Latte, 307
Lemon Ginger Gut-Restoring Tea, 306
Lemon-Lime Ginger Immunity Water, 304
Liver Love Tonic, 305
Strawberry Lemon Basil Spritzer, 304–5
Vanilla Turmeric Golden Milk Latte, 306–7
recipes, bowls and salads, 314–24
about: building bowls, 314–16; building salads, 318–20
Autumn-Inspired Salad, 322
Avocado Sauce, 316–17
Baja Bowl, 316
Buddha Bowl, 318
The Green Goddess Salad, 321
Healthy Curry Chicken Salad on Mixed Greens, 323–24

About the Author

Dr. Mariza Snyder is a functional practitioner, women's health expert, and the author of eight books, including the bestsellers *The Essential Oils Hormone Solution, The DASH Diet Cookbook,* and *Smart Mom's Guide to Essential Oils.* She has lectured at wellness centers, conferences, and corporations on hormone health, essential oils, nutrition, and detoxification. She has been featured on *The Dr. Oz Show* and Fox News Health, as well as in *O: The Oprah Magazine,* MindBodyGreen, and many other publications. Dr. Mariza is also the host of the top-rated *Essentially You* podcast, designed to empower women to become the CEO of their health. She lives with her husband and son in San Diego, California.